The IMA Volumes in Mathematics and its Applications

Volume 108

Series Editors
Willard Miller, Jr. Robert Gulliver

Springer
New York
Berlin
Heidelberg
Barcelona
Hong Kong
London
Milan
Paris
Singapore
Tokyo

Institute for Mathematics and its Applications IMA

The **Institute for Mathematics and its Applications** was established by a grant from the National Science Foundation to the University of Minnesota in 1982. The IMA seeks to encourage the development and study of fresh mathematical concepts and questions of concern to the other sciences by bringing together mathematicians and scientists from diverse fields in an atmosphere that will stimulate discussion and collaboration.

The IMA Volumes are intended to involve the broader scientific community in this process.

Willard Miller, Jr., Professor and Director

* * * * * * * * * *

IMA ANNUAL PROGRAMS

1982–1983	Statistical and Continuum Approaches to Phase Transition
1983–1984	Mathematical Models for the Economics of Decentralized Resource Allocation
1984–1985	Continuum Physics and Partial Differential Equations
1985–1986	Stochastic Differential Equations and Their Applications
1986–1987	Scientific Computation
1987–1988	Applied Combinatorics
1988–1989	Nonlinear Waves
1989–1990	Dynamical Systems and Their Applications
1990–1991	Phase Transitions and Free Boundaries
1991–1992	Applied Linear Algebra
1992–1993	Control Theory and its Applications
1993–1994	Emerging Applications of Probability
1994–1995	Waves and Scattering
1995–1996	Mathematical Methods in Material Science
1996–1997	Mathematics of High Performance Computing
1997–1998	Emerging Applications of Dynamical Systems
1998–1999	Mathematics in Biology
1999–2000	Reactive Flows and Transport Phenomena
2000–2001	Mathematics in Multi-Media

Continued at the back

Donald G. Truhlar W. Jeffrey Howe
Anthony J. Hopfinger Jeff Blaney
Richard A. Dammkoehler
Editors

Rational Drug Design

With 55 Illustrations

Springer

Donald G. Truhlar
Department of Chemistry
University of Minnesota
Minneapolis, MN 55455-0431, USA

Anthony J. Hopfinger
Department of Medicinal Chemistry
and Pharmacognocy
College of Pharmacy
University of Illinois at Chicago
Chicago, IL 60612-7231, USA

Richard A. Dammkoehler
Department of Computer Science
Washington University
St. Louis, MO 63130, USA

W. Jeffrey Howe
Unit 7247-267-1
Pharmacia & Upjohn Inc.
Kalamazoo, MI 49001, USA

Jeff Blaney
Metaphorics LLC
130 Alta Avenue
Piedmont, CA 94611, USA

Series Editors:
Willard Miller, Jr.
Robert Gulliver
Institute for Mathematics and its
Applications
University of Minnesota
Minneapolis, MN 55455, USA

Mathematics Subject Classifications (1991): 92B99, 92C40, 92B10, 82B80

Library of Congress Cataloging-in-Publication Data
Rational drug design / [edited by] Donald G. Truhlar . . . [et al.].
p. cm. — (The IMA volumes in mathematics and its
applications ; 108)
Includes bibliographical referenes.
ISBN 0-387-98753-3 (alk. paper)
1. Drugs—Design—Computer simulation—Congresses. 2. Drugs—
Design—Mathematical models—Congresses. 3. Computer-aided design—
Congresses. 4. QSAR (Biochemistry)—Congresses. I. Truhlar,
Donald G., 1944– . II. Series.
[DNLM: 1. Drug Design congresses. 2. Models, Molecular
congresses. 3. Computer Simulation congresses. QV 744 R236 1999]
RS420.R36 1999
615'.19—dc21
DNLM/DLC 98-55465

Printed on acid-free paper.

Production managed by A. Orrantia; manufacturing supervised by Nancy Wu.
Camera-ready copy prepared by the IMA.

9 8 7 6 5 4 3 2 1

ISBN 0-387-98753-3 Springer-Verlag New York Berlin Heidelberg SPIN 10709698

FOREWORD

This IMA Volume in Mathematics and its Applications

RATIONAL DRUG DESIGN

is based on the proceedings of a workshop on "Mathematical and Computational Issues in Drug Design" which was an integral part of the 1996–97 IMA program on "MATHEMATICS IN HIGH-PERFORMANCE COMPUTING." The workshop brought together top researchers in computer-aided drug discovery, computational chemistry, mathematics, and computer science to present state-of-the-art research in both the science and the underlying mathematics.

We thank Donald G. Truhlar of University of Minnesota (Chemistry and Supercomputer Institute), W. Jeffrey Howe of Pharmacia and Upjohn, Anthony J. Hopfinger of University of Illinois at Chicago (Pharmacy), Jeff Blaney of Metaphorics, and Richard A. Dammkoehler of Washington University (Computer Science) for their excellent work in organizing the workshop and editing the proceedings.

We also take this opportunity to thank the National Science Foundation (NSF), Minnesota Supercomputer Institute (MSI), and the Army Research Office (ARO), whose financial support made the workshop possible.

Willard Miller, Jr., Professor and Director

Robert Gulliver, Associate Director

PREFACE

Drug research and discovery are of critical importance in human health care and are becoming increasingly expensive, while the need for new drugs is also increasing. Computational approaches for discovery and optimization of drug leads have proven successful in many recent research programs. (A "lead" compound is one with sought for bioactivity but which requires further optimization, for example to improve its bioavailability or reduce certain side reactions, in order to become a useful drug.) Methods for drug lead discovery and optimization have grown in their effectiveness not only because of improved understanding of the basic science — the biological events and molecular interactions that define a target for therapeutic intervention — but also because of advances in algorithms, representations, and mathematical procedures for studying drug processes. In order to promote the interaction of mathematicians, computer scientists, and chemists to further the progress in the field and alert researchers to the opportunities for interdisciplinary research, the University of Minnesota's Institute for Mathematics and Its Applications and the University of Minnesota Supercomputer Institute sponsored a Workshop on Rational Drug Design on the Minneapolis campus, April 7–11, 1997. The workshop was devoted primarily to mathematical and computational issues in drug design. This volume contains the proceedings of that Workshop.

The workshop brought together top researchers in computer-aided drug discovery, computational chemistry, mathematics, and computer science to present state-of-the-art research in both the science and the underlying mathematics and to identify new problems for possible collaborations. General subject areas of the workshop included receptor-based applications such as binding energy approximations, molecular docking, and de novo design; non-receptor-based applications such as molecular similarity, conformational analysis, and structural diversity; molecular dynamics simulations; and solvation issues related to partitioning of a solute between aqueous and nonpolar media. The workshop focused on the mathematical procedures and algorithms upon which the scientific applications are based. These include graph theory and topology, non-linear multidimensional optimization, the processing and representation of information obtained from simulation studies, global optimization and search strategies, plus performance enhancement through parallel computing architectures. In addition to the oral presentations, the workshop included two panel discussions, one examining the most important current problems in drug design that may be computationally tractable, and the second focusing on emerging areas of study in which improvements in scientific knowledge over the next few years may enable the fruitful application of computational methods. The overall goal of this workshop was to bring together scientists and mathematicians to examine the current state of this very broad and interdisciplinary field of research, and to identify the areas where cross-fertilization of ideas and collaborative research might most effectively advance the field.

A broad landscape of high-profile topics in computer-assisted molecular design (CAMD) directed to drug design were covered over the course of the Workshop. Several of these topics involve finding working solutions to problems where mathematicians and mathematically oriented physical scientists might provide new direction and insight. Among the problems presented were two which permeate many fields of research today. One of these two problems is sampling high-dimensional spaces. In CAMD applications, sampling problems arise in performing conformational analysis, searching for molecular alignments, and carrying out molecular simulations. The other of these two problems is determining all extrema of a high-dimension functional interrelationship. Identification of stable states (conformations, crystal structures, and ligand-receptor binding modes) corresponds to finding minima in potential energy functions; barriers to reaction, conformational interconversion, and melt transitions correspond to saddle points. Optimum structure-activity relations correspond to extrema of penalty functions or of average deviations of prediction from experiment in correlation models.

The construction of correlation models actually presents a whole family of mathematical problems identified at the Workshop. The most direct CAMD application area in correlation model construction is quantitative structure-activity relationship (QSAR) analysis. Central to the construction of QSARs is the maximum extraction of information from data sets which are highly oversubscribed, that is, for which the number of independent variables is much greater than the number of dependent variables, as is the case for applications of comparative molecular field analysis (CoMFA). The opposite case, the number of independent variables being much less than the number of dependent variables, an undersubscribed problem, is also of concern. Here the issue is to get the most representative, robust, and reliable model from the data set.

The multiple extrema problem also arises in constructing statistical models. Data sets can contain multiple stable correlation models. There is a need to know how many distinct models are inherent to the data set and to be able to rank those models with respect to measures of significance, reliability, and robustness.

Theory can also contribute to expanding the data set by producing theoretical data to characterize potential drug molecules that have never been made. Use of force fields to determine the likely steric and electrostatic fit of a proposed molecule to a binding site is the most prominent example. An example of a frontier in this area was a paper on the use of quantum mechanical modeling to calculate charge distributions, solvation energies, and partition coefficients for small molecules.

Many of the opportunities for new mathematical contributions to this field are occasioned by the recent prominence of combinatorial libraries. Such libraries can be synthesized and assayed by robots, but mathematical modeling can play a very important role in prioritizing the targets to be made and making sense of the results. Because very large numbers of molecules can be involved, there is a new emphasis on rapidity and efficiency of the computational tools.

In a stimulating after-dinner speech at the Workshop banquet, Dr. Ralph Hirschmann of the University of Pennsylvania drew on his long industrial experience to present another perspective on drug design, focusing on many non-computational issues. For example, he discussed a 1997 paper in the *Journal of the American Chemical Society* where researchers found that the shape of a base inserted in DNA, rather than its hydrogen-bonding ability, may be the key to the polymerase recognition process that leads to faithful copying of DNA. Although this is an experimental result, by underscoring the role of 3-D shape it further dramatizes the role that computation can play in designing biotechnological molecules that mimic one or another capability of natural biological molecules. Dr. Hirschmann, however, took exception to the use of "rational drug design" and "computer-aided drug design" as near synonyms; he claims that pharmaceutical researchers were not totally irrational before they had computers! While this may be true, we hope that the Workshop and these proceedings will continue the trend of more and more productive uses of mathematical and computational techniques for the eminently humanistic goal of the design of new and better drug molecules.

Donald G. Truhlar

W. Jeffrey Howe

Anthony J. Hopfinger

Jeff Blaney

Richard A. Dammkoehler

CONTENTS

Receptor-Based Modeling

Numerical Methods

PANEL DISCUSSION: IMPORTANT CURRENT PROBLEMS IN DRUG DESIGN THAT MAY BE COMPUTATIONALLY TRACTABLE

Panelists: DAVE DOHERTY[1], BILL DUNN[2] GRAHAM RICHARDS[3], and DOUG ROHRER[4]

Moderators: A.J. HOPFINGER[2] and W.J. HOWE[5]

The intent of the first panel discussion was to identify areas, within the broad range of fields represented at the workshop, in which there are particularly important problems that may be amenable to theoretical, mathematical, or computational advancement. The focus was on areas that are currently under study, as opposed to the second panel discussion which covered areas that one may anticipate will begin to yield to computational methods within 5–10 years or so. Given the breadth of the subject matter covered at the workshop, the issues presented during the panel discussions were necessarily only a small subset of a potential list of "important problems," and they were obviously biased by the particular areas of research interest of the panelists. Nonetheless, each of the issues presented by a panelist engendered considerable discussion among the workshop participants, and the issues discussed in the first panel session can be considered to be representative of problems currently under study by numerous scientists in the field.

The panel discussion was structured around brief presentations by each of the panelists on one or more issues viewed as particularly difficult or important for the furtherance of the field. Each presentation was then followed by discussion among the larger audience. After the four presentations were complete, additional topics and issues were put forth for discussion by workshop participants. Following is a brief summary of the issues presented by the panelists and other participants.

The approach taken by Graham Richards was to present the drug discovery process as a continuum — an essentially linear process that begins with genes, and moves through proteins of therapeutic interest that are

[1]Minnesota Supercomputer Center, Inc., 1200 Washington Avenue South, Minneapolis, MN 55415.

[2]Deparment of Medicinal Chemistry and Pharmacognocy, University of Illinois at Chicago, College of Pharmacy, 833 South Wood Street, Chicago, IL 60612-7231.

[3]Physical Chemistry Laboratory, Oxford University, South Parks Road, Oxford OX1, 3QZ, United Kingdom.

[4]Computer-Aided Drug Discovery, Pharmacia and Upjohn, Inc., 301 Henrietta St., Kalamazoo, MI 49007–4940.

[5]Unit 7247–267–1, Pharmacia and Upjohn, 301 Henrietta St., Kalamazoo, MI 49001.

encoded by the genes, to small molecules (potential drugs) that are designed to modulate the function of the target proteins. At the genetic end, the problem most suited to computing (and particularly, supercomputing) is hunting for sequence similarities between known genes and the entire genome database. The vast amount of data from sequencing the human genome and those of pathogens means that this is an enormous computational task. A recent example of the types of discoveries that can be made from such data mining is the identification of the similarity between smallpox viral genes and some of the genes in the human immunodefense system. It is clear at this point that the rapidly increasing amount of genetic data that are becoming available, coupled with the increasing reliance of pharmaceutical companies on the selection of drug targets based on information contained in these databases, will translate to substantial opportunities for improvements in bioinformatics algorithms.

Moving along the continuum, the greatest scientific challenge remains the 'protein folding problem' — going from gene sequence (and therefore protein sequence) to protein structure. Sequence identification far outpaces experimental structure solution, so there is a need to predict structure from sequence. Folding must depend on sequence and physics, but new insights and methods are needed. This remains the "Nobel Prize" problem.

Moving from protein targets to the small molecules that are being designed to bind to them, it is noted that such molecules are increasingly being synthesized by combinatorial or highly parallel synthesis techniques. While such methods are able to generate molecules on a scale of tens to hundreds of thousands, there is a need (and a recent trend) to reduce the structure space somewhat by clever application of computational methods to achieve greater focus and to improve the odds of identifying active compounds. This also carries over to the need for more efficient methods for comparing and selecting molecules (with specified properties) from databases containing hundreds of thousands of "real" compounds, to billions of "virtual" compounds (currently existing databases), each of which can have many conformationally-accessible structures. It was noted in the workshop that organic structure-space, of molecular weight less than 500, has been estimated variously as from 10^{60} to 10^{400} unique compounds.

Doug Rohrer's focus was in the "small molecule" region of the continuum. He noted that many of the current challenges in making sense of structure-activity relation (SAR) data relate to choices, and that a large number of choices are generally required. To name a few, these choices range from selection of compounds, generating 3D structures for each compound (the conformational flexibility problem), determining the most appropriate overlay of the compounds (alignment rules), defining a consensus multi-molecule binding model, and determining how the consensus features of the model can best be used in drug discovery and optimization (that is, now that we have a model, what do we do with it?).

The initial choice of compounds used to develop an SAR model typically encompasses a small number of highest-affinity compounds. However, as the project matures, the selection of additional compounds must include as much diversity as possible, in both the 2D (connectivity) and 3D (spatial) sense. The challenge is to evaluate this diversity quickly. It is important, as was mentioned numerous times during the workshop, to maintain a fast turn-around time on such studies in order to remain in the decision and design loops. Otherwise the chemistry will move ahead without it. Doug suggested that perhaps improved graph theoretic approaches could be applied at this stage.

Usually the compounds of interest can have numerous low energy conformations. The challenges here involve methods for exploring conformational space, followed by analysis to select a representative subset of diverse conformations. Several novel methods were presented at the workshop which may address this challenge. One involved reducing the 3D structures to a 2D format that retains more information than does a simple projection technique. Modifications of alphanumeric character recognition algorithms were then used to identify similar shapes. Another technique that was presented involved mapping the structures into pre-defined arrangements of spheres to classify the shape of the molecules. Such classification of the molecular shape could provide a starting point for the production of multiple molecule overlays to generate the SAR model.

Field-based similarity matching provides an excellent means of optimizing structural overlays. However, the speed of this process needs to be improved in order to be useful with larger numbers of molecules (greater than ten). In addition, information about the relative biological potencies somehow needs to be factored into this process, so that the good, the bad, and the ugly features of the overlay model can be identified.

Finally, methods to use the overlay features of the SAR model to derive new molecules algorithmically, to test hand-generated molecules against the model, or to optimize existing leads via suggestions from the model, would be the ultimate goals. Automated *de novo* design programs like GROWMOL might be a start, but the solution is still elusive.

Bill Dunn continued the discussion of challenges related to small-molecule design, and again, for the common situation where the 3D structure of the target (protein) is not known, leading to the application of indirect methods in the delineation of 3D quantitative structure-activity relations (QSAR). One difficulty with these methodologies (e.g. comparative molecular field analysis, molecular shape analysis, etc.) is the assignment of a receptor-bound conformation (conformational flexibility again) and an alignment for the ligands (overlay problem). This is generally done by trial and error, with some guidance provided by ligands with restricted degrees of conformational freedom. This is an extremely costly exercise that limits the utility of 3D-QSAR.

A general solution to this problem may be found by relaxing the conformation and alignment constraints of existing approaches, and by describing the active ligands with features that vary with conformation and alignment. The resulting arrays are third-order tensors that can be decomposed to yield the descriptor vector(s) most highly correlated with biological activity.

Dunn's group is exploring a general formalism for 3D-QSAR that includes various methods useful for the decomposition of 3-way arrays of conformation- and alignment-dependent feature data. They are also exploring novel methods of aligning sets of bioactive compounds, in such a way that leads to an unconstrained 3D-QSAR procedure.

Dave Doherty focused on problems in biological chemistry that are characterized by structural transitions that involve large-scale motions of portions of the structure. One obvious example of this is the folding of proteins. But there are other, less global, changes that also occur via large scale motions, and Doherty's statement of the problem of identifying these transitions was aimed at discovering cooperative or nonlinear effects that cause such large scale motions. Definitive answers to these questions would contribute greatly to our understanding of protein structure, and particularly to our ability to predict tertiary structure and its longer time-scale behavior.

The issues that he raised were intended to provoke thought among the mathematicians and drug designers about how further improvements in solutions to nonlinear mathematical systems might shed some light on current problems in drug design. To motivate such thought, an example was given of some of his studies that used direct molecular dynamics simulation to search for nonlinear motions that have long been postulated to be characteristic of the so-called "rotator" pre-melting phases in *n*-paraffin crystals (Doherty, D. C., Hopfinger, A. J., *Phys. Rev. Lett.* (1994) **72** (5), 661). These "sine-Gordon" soliton waves arise from the solutions to a set of nonlinear differential equations. The fact that these equations have an analytical solution (a traveling arctangent waveform) provides a unique opportunity to search for these cooperative motions using direct simulation. This work appears to have definitively identified these high amplitude, localized waves in the molecular dynamics simulations, even though there is no explicit term in the molecular mechanics force field that specifically gives rise to them — which is indicative of the cooperative effects of a collection of multiple chains.

This is an exciting development in our understanding of cooperative effects in molecular phase transitions. So, to the attending mathematicians one might ask, "What are the current developments in solutions (analytical or simulated) to molecular dynamics equations for complex systems that may be of some use in our understanding of cooperative processes in biochemical systems?" And one might ask the computational chemists, "What are the important questions that might move us along to a better understanding of cooperative effects, through some combination of mathematics and direct simulation?"

After the panelists' presentations and the ensuing discussions, additional challenges were put forth by other workshop participants. It was noted that few of the issues discussed to that point related to what has become known as 'direct methods' — techniques such as docking, *de novo* design, ligand-binding scoring, and so on, that can be applied when the target protein is known in structural detail. Such detailed knowledge is becoming much more common, in part because of the rapid emergence of genomics-based targets. In many pharmaceutical companies, all new discovery programs are molecularly-based, and they follow the continuum outlined by Graham Richards. Genomics is used to select the target, which is then further developed through cloning, expression, folding, and purification of the relevant protein(s) to produce molecular (and generally, high throughput) assays of small-molecule activity. With protein on hand, structural biology (X-ray crystallography, NMR structure determination, antibody epitope mapping, and so on) can provide the structural detail needed for application of direct methods to the task of lead discovery, or at least to lead optimization. (An "epitope" is the surface region of another molecule that is recognized and bound by an antibody. A "lead" is a compound with the sought for bioactivity, but which requires further optimization, for example to improve its bioavailability or eliminate certain side reactions, in order to become a useful drug.)

A number of the important issues in this area were discussed in the main workshop presentations during the week. One of the most pressing issues was improved methods for dealing with the physics and physical chemistry of water, sometimes through explicit consideration of solvation effects during simulations or binding energy calculations, but more typically through continuum solvation models. It was stated by one of the participants that we can generally do quite well now in predicting geometries of potential drug molecules at a binding site, but not so well in accounting for their solvation effects on the binding energy or even for the intrinsic components of the binding energy. Accurate calculation of ligand/protein binding energies (including entropic considerations) was generally viewed as one of the most important current needs, as it pervades all of the direct-methods techniques for studying and predicting the activity of small-molecule analogs. It was also noted that, in order to remain within the design cycle, molecular modelers must choose their methods, in part, on the basis of speed, to provide quick turn-around of results. This places a greater burden on finding energy-based methods or scoring functions that are accurate and *fast*. The need for speed is most evident in the effective application of automated *de novo* design methods, where tens to hundreds of thousands of candidate structures must be generated, evaluated (by some form of scoring function which assesses goodness of fit to the target), and assigned a priority ranking. Of course, when opting for methods that are fast, one must always question whether the reliability of the results warrants the use of the faster methods.

Another participant went further and pointed out that many of the currently available methods typically produce huge lists of seemingly reasonable molecules. However, only a few can be chosen for synthesis. Ideally a free energy scoring function would provide a basis for ranking and selecting the structures. Despite much progress, this remains an unsolved problem. Although the list can be reduced, one cannot with confidence pick only the top ten or so compounds for further study. Until the perfect scoring function is developed one must sample the reduced list in some rational manner. Experimental design methods are needed to address this. This is an opportunity for closer collaboration between the computational chemistry community and the statistical and applied mathematics community.

PANEL DISCUSSION: NEW PROBLEMS THAT SHOULD BE ADDRESSED IN THE NEXT TEN YEARS

Panelists: GORDON CRIPPEN[1], SIMON KEARSLEY[2], GARLAND MARSHALL[3] and PHIL PORTOGHESE[4]

Moderator: JEFF BLANEY[5]

This panel's challenge was to identify important problems and challenges in drug discovery that should be addressed within the next decade given steady, predictable improvement in computational power and perhaps less predictable improvement in algorithms and methods. What are the pressing problems and bottlenecks that may succumb to new computational and theoretical approaches?

Garland Marshall discussed the need for improved methods to deal with error analysis and propagation of errors in the drug discovery and optimization process. We routinely face many sources of error, experimental and theoretical, that complicate our efforts to interpret and predict structure-activity relationships. He also noted that we need to improve our ability to predict the structure of drug receptors. Despite the impressive increases in the ability of Xray crystallography and NMR to solve the structures of biologically relevant macromolecules, many critical receptors remain intractable. For example, 7-helical transmembrane, G protein-coupled receptors (7TM GPCRs) make up the largest single class of receptor targeted by today's drugs, yet no experimental structures are available due to the extreme difficulties in crystallizing transmembrane proteins. He also noted the immense informatics problem posed by the explosion of data available on the internet. We're "drowning in a sea of data," with only primitive tools to integrate, assimilate, and interpret the data. The explosion of genomics data is only beginning, due to the massive efforts behind the human genome project (the goal is to completely sequence the 3 billion bases in human DNA by 2005) and other sequencing efforts targeting a variety of microorganisms and pathogens.

Phil Portoghese also discussed the importance of 7TM GPCRs, noting that our only structural information comes from low-resolution experimental data and approximate homology models. The mechanism by which 7TM GPCRs transduce an extracellular signal across the membrane is poorly understood. He described experimental methods that can provide additional

[1]College of Pharmacy, University of Michigan, Ann Arbor, Michigan 48109-1065.

[2]Merck Research Laboratorles, PO Box 2000, Rahway, NJ 07065.

[3]Center for Molecular Design, Washington Unlversity, St. Louis, MO 63130–4899.

[4]College of Pharmacy, University of Minnesota, 8-111 WDH, 308 Harvard Street SE, Minneapolis, MN 55455.

[5]Metaphorics, 130 Alta Avenue, Pledmont, CA 94611.

data to help modeling, such as recent work in making chimeric receptors that combine features of two different receptors in a single molecule. For example, an extracellular loop of the kappa-opiate receptor was transferred to the mu-opiate receptor, resulting in a new, kappa-selective, chimeric receptor. Current structures and models are not able to explain the difference between 7TM GPCR agonists (molecules that turn on an intracellular response) and antagonists (molecules that inhibit the intracellular response). For example, morphine-type molecules containing an N-CH_3 group are agonists at the mu-opiate receptor, but converting the N-CH_3 group to N-CH_2-cyclopropyl produces an antagonist. This is a very small structural change, yet it produces a dramatically different response.

Gordon Crippen noted that structure-activity relationships and computer-assisted drug design rely on the rather vague notion of molecular similarity as a central theme: similar molecules tend to have similar biological activity. However, we have many different ways of defining, measuring, and calculating similarity. He suggested that molecular similarity should be defined relative to the environment in which it is being measured, rather than as an independent property. He also addressed the critical problem of modeling oral bioavailability and drug distribution within the body. We have extremely limited control and understanding of how to alter chemical structure to achieve the desired properties (for example, a pill that is stable in the gut, reaches the target organ and receptors intact, has a long enough half-life to require only 1–2 doses per day, and does not produce toxic metabolites). Drug design and discovery is a complex, interdisciplinary problem: rather than focus on isolated problems, we should consider the entire system as a large graph depicting how drugs interact with the body. The nodes are organs, tissues, fluids, membranes, and other structures within the body. The edges are known or hypothetical pathways; sometimes there may be more than one path between a pair of nodes. Nodes are labeled by various capacities, edges by rates and permissions. Can we integrate known data into such a model?

Simon Kearsley provided a brief historical overview and a map to the future of modeling challenges, noting that modeling has already had a large impact in lead identification and optimization. Due to the advent of high-throughput screening, genomics, and bioinformatics, data mining and modeling are being used to help biologists get needed chemistry support (for example, by computationally identifying existing molecules in databases that validate biological hypotheses, which in turn creates demand for additional, optimized molecules). Current approaches have focused on the early stages of drug discovery by improving the odds through statistical and qualititative methods, for example, by helping to prioritize screening and assisting in the identification of new leads. Such methods include two-dimensional chemical substructure and similarity searching, and three-dimensional superposition and docking calculations. He suggested that the next challenge is in information science: extrapolating from data mining to "concept" mining and mining relationships in the data, going beyond improving the odds by studying case histories and anticipating decision points. He also mentioned that modeling approaches will need to head toward modeling cellular processes and relationships (similar to Gordon Crippen's ideas). This will require a canonicalization of text, and the building of regular vocabularies and thesauri to deal with the huge number of imprecise names and synonyms in biology. A formalized mathematical language will need to be developed for biology which can deal with a limited number of observable properties and data. He mentioned the need for technology to deal with very large databases and "data warehousing": for example, data integration, data "scrubbing," and multidimensional trend analysis. He also discussed the need for rule-generating algorithms that can deal with fuzzy logic and ambiguity. These methods will need to define and measure information content, including the subjectivity content, deal with noise and sparse data, and capture human expertise and knowledge.

There are clearly huge problems, challenges, and opportunities for drug discovery in the next decade. Most of today's methods focus on the early phases of drug discovery, which consume only a small fraction of the time and money (less than 20%) of the total path (10–12 years, \$300–500 million) on the way to a marketed drug. Integrated approaches such as those suggested by Kearsley and Crippen have the potential to improve drug discovery further down the expensive and time-consuming development process, but will require increasingly sophisticated computational methods and information science technology.

MATCHING OF CHEMICAL AND BIOLOGICAL STRUCTURES USING SUBGRAPH AND MAXIMAL COMMON SUBGRAPH ISOMORPHISM ALGORITHMS

PETER WILLETT*

Abstract. This paper discusses the use of graph-isomorphism algorithms for substructure and maximal common substructure searching in databases of chemical and biological molecules. Subgraph isomorphism algorithms are used in substructure searching, where one wishes to identify all molecules in a database that contain a user-defined pattern, with an initial screening search being used to eliminate a large fraction of the database from the time-consuming graph-matching search. A maximal common subgraph isomorphism algorithm provides an effective way of identifying the structural features common to a pair of molecules. The application of these isomorphism techniques to database searching is illustrated by reference to 2D and 3D small molecules, 3D protein structures and carbohydrate sequences.

Key words. ASSAM, Carbohydrate sequence, Complex Carbohydrate Structure Database, Connection table, Database searching, DISCO, Field-graph, Graph theory, Maximal common subgraph isomorphism, Molecular electrostatic potential, Pharmacophore mapping, Pharmacophoric pattern matching, Protein Data Bank, Protein structure, PROTEP, Similarity searching, Subgraph isomorphism, Substructure searching

1. Chemical graphs. Modern pharmaceutical research is making increasing use of sophisticated information systems that allow the storage and the retrieval of chemical structural information (Ash *et al.*, 1991; Good and Mason, 1996; Martin and Willett, 1997). These systems are based on long-established methods for the processing of two-dimensional (2D) chemical structure diagrams (Morgan, 1965; Ray and Kirsch, 1957; Sussenguth, 1965) that derive from the branch of mathematics known as *graph theory* (Trinajstic, 1983; Wilson, 1972). A *graph* describes a set of objects, called *nodes* or *vertices*, and the relationships, called *edges* or *arcs*, that exist between pairs of these objects. Graph theory covers many different characteristics of graphs: here, we focus on the *isomorphism* techniques that have been developed for establishing the structural relationships that exist between pairs of graphs (Gati, 1979; McGregor, 1982; Read and Corneil, 1977). Specifically, we discuss the use of such techniques for matching the graphs representing a query (sub)structure and one of the structures in a database that is to be searched.

A graph, G, consists of a set of nodes together with a set of edges connecting pairs of nodes, and two nodes are said to be *adjacent* if they are connected by an edge. Two graphs, G_1 and G_2, are *isomorphic* if there is an exact correspondence between the nodes of G_1 and of G_2 such that adjacent pairs of nodes in G_1 are mapped to adjacent pairs of nodes in G_2,

*Krebs Institute for Biomolecular Research and Department of Information Studies, University of Sheffield, Western Bank, Sheffield S10 2TN, United Kingdom. P.WILLETT@SHEFFIELD.AC.UK

i.e., if the two graphs are identical. A *subgraph* of G is a subset, P, of the nodes of G together with a subset of the edges connecting pairs of nodes in P. A *subgraph isomorphism* exists if G_1 is a subgraph of G_2 (or *vice versa*) and a *subgraph-isomorphism algorithm* is thus a computational procedure that determines whether one graph is a subgraph of another. Finally, a *common subgraph* of two graphs G_1 and G_2 is defined as consisting of a subgraph g_1 of G_1 and a subgraph g_2 of G_2 such that g_1 is isomorphic to g_2; the *maximal common subgraph* (or MCS) is the largest such common subgraph. A graph is said to be *labelled* if identifier labels are associated with the nodes and/or edges, and it is said to be *directed* if each of the edges specifies not only that a relationship exists between a pair of nodes but also the direction of that relationship. All of the types of graph considered in this paper are labelled and the carbohydrate graphs discussed in Section 3 are also directed.

A graph provides a natural machine-readable representation of a 2D chemical structure diagram. Such a representation, which is normally referred to as a *connection table*, contains a list of all of the (usually non-hydrogen) atoms within a structure, together with bond information that describes the exact manner in which the individual atoms are linked together. A database of 2D chemical structures can hence be represented by a file of labelled graphs, with these being processed by one of the isomorphism procedures mentioned in the previous paragraph to support one of the important search functions in a chemical information system. *Structure searching* involves determining whether two chemical compounds are identical (as would be required, for example, when one needed to search a database to find the biological activity data associated with a specific query molecule) and is effected by means of a graph isomorphism algorithm (Ash *et al.*, 1991). Substructure searching involves determining whether a database structure contains a query substructure (such as a specific ring system) and is effected by means of a subgraph isomorphism algorithm (Barnard, 1993). *Similarity searching* is an alternative means of accessing a chemical database in which a *target* molecule of interest, such as a weak lead from a high-throughput screening programme, is matched against all of the molecules in a database to find the *nearest neighbours*, *i.e.*, those molecules that are most similar to the target using some quantitative measure of inter-molecular similarity (Downs and Willett, 1996). One way in which this can be done is to use the largest substructure common to a pair of structures as the similarity measure, and this is effected by means of an MCS algorithm.

Such graph-based matching procedures have been used for many years to process 2D small molecules, but it is only recently that it has been realised that graph-theoretic techniques are also applicable to the processing of three-dimensional (3D) structures and biological macromolecules. A continuing programme of research in the University of Sheffield is exploring such applications, and the present paper provides a review of this work to date.

2. Chemical substructure searching. The relationship between a graph and a connection table means that a subgraph isomorphism algorithm can be used to determine whether the connection table representing a query substructure is contained within the connection table representing a database structure. This forms the basis of substructure searching, or *atom-by-atom* searching, which was first described by Ray and Kirsch (1957) some four decades ago and which is still probably the most important facility offered within a chemical information system.

Substructure searching is normally implemented by means of a backtracking, depth-first tree search. This involves matching a pair of atoms (one from the query substructure and one from a database structure) and then attempting to match their neighbours. If the neighbours can be matched then the process is repeated for their neighbours; alternatively, if a match is not obtained, then it is undone and another possible mapping tried. The procedure terminates when the complete set of query atoms (and hence the entire query substructure) has been matched or when every possible mapping has been tried. Improvements in performance can be achieved using *relaxation* techniques. Relaxation involves assigning a value to a node and then iteratively refining it by examining the values of neighbouring nodes; at each stage, a note is made of those nodes in the matching structure that have equal values. This procedure results in a database structure and a query substructure being iteratively partitioned into sets of potentially-matching nodes, thus reducing the numbers of comparisons that need to be made during the subsequent backtracking search. Detailed comparisons of several different subgraph isomorphism algorithms (Brint and Willett, 1987a; Downs *et al.*, 1988) suggest that the algorithm due to Ullmann (1976) is the most appropriate for substructure searching. The Ullmann algorithm starts by invoking a relaxation technique to provide an initial set of matching nodes and then proceeds with a depth-first backtrack search. At each step of the search, as a potential match is made, the relaxation procedure is invoked again, thus further reducing the amount of backtracking that is required.

Subgraph isomorphism belongs to a class of computational problems that are referred to as *NP-complete* (Garey and Johnson, 1979) and that are known to be extremely demanding of computational resources. Substructure searching involves determining the presence or absence of a subgraph isomorphism between the query substructure and each and every one of the molecules in a database, and it will thus be extremely time-consuming unless efficient search algorithms and substantial computing power are available. These computational problems are lessened to some extent, in that the graphs stored in 2D chemical information systems are far simpler than those considered in many applications of graph theory, since both the nodes and the edges here are labelled (with the elemental and bond types, respectively) and since the graphs are of low connectivity (since each node is linked to only a small number of other nodes). Even so, there has been much interest in techniques that can minimise the computational costs of substructure searching in large databases (Ash *et al.*, 1991).

The principal strategy that has been adopted is to use an initial *screen search*, where a screen is a substructural feature, the presence of which is necessary, but not sufficient, for a molecule to contain the query substructure. These features are typically small, atom-, bond- or ring-centred fragment substructures that are algorithmically generated from a connection table when a molecule is added to the database that is to be searched. Fragments differ considerably in their discriminatory abilities, and algorithmic methods have thus been developed to identify a subset of all of the possible fragments that will maximise screenout in substructure searches. These studies suggest that the most useful fragments for screening purposes are those of intermediate, and approximately equal, frequencies of occurrence in the database that is to be searched (see, *e.g.*, Cringean *et al.*, 1990; Hodes, 1976). The fragments that have been chosen to comprise the *screenset*, *i.e.*, the set of fragments that are to be used for screening, are listed in a fragment coding dictionary. When a query substructure or a database structure is to be processed, the corresponding connection table is analysed to identify those screens from the coding dictionary that are present in the structure. The input (sub)structure is then represented by a fixed-length bit-string, in which the non-zero bits correspond to the screens that are present. These bit-strings form the basis for the screen search, which is effected by checking each of the database structures for the presence of the screens that are present in the query substructure. Alternatively, *fingerprint*-based approaches replace the idea of a screenset by the enumeration and encoding of all fragments within a molecule, using a superimposed coding scheme to create the query and database bit-strings (Barnard, 1993).

A screen can be regarded as being analogous to an entry in an index, in that it provides access to that subset of the database that contains some particular characteristic. It is thus to be expected that only a very small fraction of the search file will contain all of the screens that have been assigned to the query substructure. It is these few molecules that are passed on for the final, time-consuming atom-by-atom search, which ensures that there is an exact subgraph isomorphism between the graphs representing the query substructure and the database structure. The simple, two-stage procedure (*i.e.*, screen searching and geometric searching) described above has formed the basis for many operational 2D substructure searching systems, although other approaches have been described in the literature (Barnard, 1993).

3. Carbohydrate substructure searching. We have recently started to investigate the application of the 2D substructure searching methodology described in the previous section to the carbohydrate molecules in the

Complex Carbohydrate Structure Database (CCSD) (Doubet *et al.*, 1989; Feizi and Bundle, 1996). This is an increasingly important resource for carbohydrate research and comes with a search program, called CarbBank, that uses pattern-matching routines to identify substrings of residues, exact matches and chains with some minimum number of residues in common. While these routines are efficient in operation, their basis in algorithms for matching sequences means that problems can arise because of the branched natures of many complex carbohydrates. Such problems can, however, be easily removed if one notes that a carbohydrate structure can be regarded as a labelled, directed graph, in which the nodes of the graph denote the individual monosaccharides and the edges denote the glycosidic linkages (Bruno *et al.*, 1997). More specifically, the root (or type) of each monosaccharide is given a three-letter abbreviation, *e.g.*, glucose and fructose are represented by Glc and Fru, respectively. These node labels are augmented by the inclusion of information concerning the ring size and the anomeric and absolute configurations. Glycosidic linkages are represented as being from one particular point on a monosaccharide to another, and each edge in a carbohydrate graph thus has an associated direction.

The availability of a connection-table representation means that it is possible to use simple modifications of the screening and subgraph-isomorphism techniques used for 2D substructure searching to search the CCSD to identify all of the carbohydrates that contain a user-defined pattern of residues and inter-residue linkages (Bruno *et al.*, 1997). Our experiments have used a file of 33,174 sequences from the most recent release of the CCSD database, with each such sequence being characterised by a 128-member screenset generated using the algorithm of Cringean *et al.* (1990). This screenset uses fragments called *augmented residues*, where an augmented residue consists of a residue together with the residues directly linked to it. These screens are used as a precursor to the subsequent *residue-by-residue* search, which involves a suitably modified implementation of the Ullmann subgraph isomorphism algorithm. An extensive series of experiments with a PC-based, Fortran 77 implementation of these ideas has shown that the screen search results in a mean screenout of 89%, thus enabling the overall search times to be comparable with those required using the established CarbBank Version 3.0 routines (in fact, about 90% of the overall search time for our searches is taken up with reading in the connection tables for those sequences that need to undergo the final residue-by-residue search).

Substructure searching in the CCSD using the CarbBank program requires that a series of *residue+complexes* must be specified and linked using Boolean operators to form a query. A residue+complex is defined as a "core" residue plus linkages to other residues and information about the attached groups, and is thus analogous to the augmented-residue screens described above. Searches using this method can lead to mismatches or *false-drops* when a structure is retrieved containing each specified residue+complex, but not connected in the manner described by the query substructure. Such erroneous retrievals do not occur in the graph-based searches owing to the inclusion of the final, residue-by-residue search.

We have found that false-drops occur quite extensively in practice. For example, in a series of 30 low-precision searches in which no account was taken of anomeric configuration, absolute configuration and ring form, 20 searches gave the same number of hits with both CarbBank and our methods, but CarbBank gave a total of 57 false-drops in the remaining 10 searches; there were still 26 such false-drops in high-precision searches in which account was taken of the three types of feature. An analysis of the search outputs demonstrates, hardly surprisingly, that the incidence of false-drops in the CarbBank searches is greater the larger the structures that are being searched. We would thus expect that the differences in search performance between the two approaches will tend to increase as more complex structures start to be included in CCSD.

4. Pharmacophoric pattern matching. Carbohydrate sequences are analogous to conventional chemical structure diagrams in that they consider only the 2D structure of a molecule, and take no account of its 3D nature. However, graph-based methods are equally applicable to the searching of such geometric representations, as first noted by Gund (1977). He suggested that the nodes and edges of a graph could be used to represent the atoms and inter-atomic distances, respectively, in a small molecule, and that the resulting inter-atomic distance matrix could then be inspected for the presence of a query *pharmacophore*, or *pharmacophoric pattern, i.e.*, the arrangement of structural features in 3D space necessary for a molecule to bind at an active site. Given that a 3D structure can be represented by a graph, the presence or absence of a pharmacophoric pattern can be confirmed by means of a subgraph isomorphism procedure in which the edges in a database structure and a query substructure are matched if they denote the same inter-atomic distance (to within any user-specified tolerance). In what follows, we shall refer to such a search as a *geometric search* to differentiate it from the atom-by-atom and residue-by-residue searches mentioned previously.

Simple pharmacophoric patterns consist of atoms, typically hydrogen donors or acceptors, together with some or all of the associated inter-atomic distances, and it thus seems natural to base a screening system on distance information. Distance is a continuous variable that can take an arbitrarily large number of values, depending upon the accuracy of the atomic co-ordinate data from which it is generated, and screens for pharmacophore searching are thus based on *ranges* of inter-atomic distances. Fragments consisting of pairs of atoms and a single distance are most common (Cringean *et al.*, 1990; Jakes and Willett, 1986; Sheridan *et al.*, 1989), but there have also been reports of the use of atom-triplets (Fisanick *et al.*, 1992; Nilakantan *et al.*, 1993) and of valence or torsion angles (Poirrette *et al.*, 1991, 1993) for database searching.

The screens that are used for 3D substructure searching thus consist of two, three or four points and an associated distance range or angular range. A database structure or query substructure is encoded by generating each fragment (*e.g.*, a pair of points and the inter-atomic distance) in turn, and then searching the screenset to identify a set of matching points and a range that includes the value occurring in the fragment. Once the screen has been identified, the appropriate location is set in the bit-string that is used for the screen search, which is implemented in much the same way as a 2D substructure search. The detailed geometric search is then invoked only for those database structures that match the query at the screen level.

The atom-by-atom level is needed in 2D substructure searching since a molecule possessing all of the query screens may still not match the query because the substructural features corresponding to these screens are connected in a different way from the pattern of linkages in the query. There is a similar problem in 3D searching, since the screens describe only the fact that the query screens are present, without taking account of the relative geometric orientations of the sets of points in 3-D space. In fact, there is a further problem with 3-D screens, in that they refer to ranges, and not to precise values; a structure may thus be assigned a query screen even though it does not contain the precise value (or range of values) for some distance or angle that has been specified in the query pharmacophore. The initial stage of a geometric search thus involves checking that the actual query values (to within any allowed tolerances) are present in the database structure that is under consideration. A molecule that passes this check then undergoes the final subgraph-isomorphism check to determine whether or not the query pharmacophore is present; if a match is obtained, then the matching atoms (or sets of atoms if multiple isomorphisms are present) are noted, *e.g.*, for subsequent input to a structure display or modelling program. The geometric search is normally effected by means of the Ullmann algorithm (Brint and Willett, 1987a; Sheridan *et al.*, 1989).

The screening and geometric searching algorithms described above provide an effective and an efficient means of access to files of 3D structures, and such techniques have enabled many pharmacophore-searching systems to be developed over the last few years (Good and Mason, 1996; Warr and Willett, 1997). However, such systems do have a major limitation in that they store only a single low-energy conformation (or a limited number of such conformations) for each molecule in a database, these conformations being either the output of an X-ray experiment or calculated using an automatic model builder (Sadowski and Gasteiger, 1993). Accordingly, a pharmacophore search is likely to miss large numbers of matching molecules that can adopt a conformation containing the query pattern but that are represented in the database by a low-energy conformation that does not contain this pattern. In what follows, 3D search systems that operate upon single conformations will be referred to as *rigid-searching* systems, and those that encompass multiple conformations as *flexible-searching* systems.

Two main approaches to flexible searching have been described. In the first, a flexible molecule is represented by some small number of carefully selected low-energy conformations, with a rigid- searching algorithm being applied to each of the conformations describing a molecule. This approach has many advantages (Warr and Willett, 1997) but it does mean that the search algorithm cannot explore the full conformational space available to a flexible molecule, with the possibility of a loss in recall. Our work in Sheffield has thus focused upon the development of algorithms and data structures that avoid such retrieval failures.

In a rigid 3D molecule, the distance between each and every pair of atoms is a single, fixed value, whereas the distance between a pair of atoms in a flexible molecule will depend on the conformation that is adopted. The separation of a pair of atoms is hence conveniently described by a *distance range*, the lowerbounds and upperbounds of which correspond to the minimum- and maximum-possible distances (though for some pairs of atoms, *e.g.*, those within an aromatic ring system, these two distances will be the same whatever conformation is adopted by the molecule). The set of distance ranges for a molecule will contain all of the geometrically-feasible conformations which that molecule can adopt, and thus provides an obvious way of representing a flexible molecule. Such sets of distance ranges can be generated using the bounds-smoothing technique that forms an important component of the *distance-geometry* approach to structure generation (Crippen and Havel, 1988).

The screening and geometric-searching algorithms that are used for rigid 3D searching operate on graphs where each edge denotes a single value; these algorithms require only minor modifications to enable them to process graphs in which each edge contains both a lowerbound and an upperbound, thus allowing the retrieval of all molecules that could possibly adopt a conformation that contains a query pharmacophoric pattern (Clark *et al.*, 1992). Indeed, it is possible to view the algorithms described previously for rigid searching as limiting cases of the more general algorithms that are required for flexible searching. There is, however, one major difference between flexible 3D and both 2D and rigid 3D substructure searching, in that those molecules that match the query in the geometric search must then undergo a further, and final, check that uses some form of conformational-searching procedure (Leach, 1991); this is required since bounds-smoothing is known to over-estimate the true range of possible inter-atomic distances. A range of methods for this final *conformational search* have been described (Clark *et al.*, 1994), of which the most effective and most efficient would seem to be a technique known as *directed tweak* (Hurst, 1994).

The techniques that have been described here are playing an increasingly important role in lead-discovery programmes for novel pharmaceutical and agrochemical compounds, typically in conjunction with a molecular modelling system. The integration of these two types of technique is very important. Modelling (either manually or *via* the pharmacophore mapping procedures described in Section 6) is most obviously used to suggest the initial pharmacophore pattern for a database search but can also be used to compare each hit with the known actives to see whether the former contain features that could destroy bioactivity, *e.g.*, the presence of other groups that might prevent the molecules from fitting into the binding site or might cause unfavourable electrostatic interactions. Such observations can help to set priorities for testing of the compounds and can suggest other analogues for synthesis that have a better chance for success. The integration of modelling and pharmacophore searching is reviewed by Bures (1997).

5. Protein substructure searching. The final application of subgraph-isomorphism algorithms to be discussed here is their use for searching 3D protein structures in the Brookhaven Protein Data Bank, PDB (Bernstein *et al.*, 1977). Two types of patterns are considered: patterns of *secondary structure elements* in 3D and patterns of *amino acid sidechains* in 3D, these being searched for using the programs PROTEP and ASSAM, respectively. In both cases, a graph representation was developed to characterise the protein structures, and the Ullmann algorithm modified to process these representations. Note that we have not felt it necessary, thus far, to develop an initial screening stage owing to the limited number of proteins for which a 3D structure is available.

5.1. Searching protein secondary structure elements. The graph representation of a protein that we have adopted for PROTEP makes use of the fact that the two most common types of secondary structure element (SSE), the α-helix and the β-strand, are both approximately linear, repeating structures, which can hence be represented by vectors drawn along their major axes. The set of vectors corresponding to the SSEs in a protein can then be used to describe that proteins 3D structure, with the SSEs and the inter-element angles and distances corresponding to the nodes and to the edges, respectively, of a graph (Mitchell *et al.*, 1990). More precisely, each edge in such a graph is a three-part data element that contains the angle between a pair of vectors describing SSEs, the distance of closest approach of the two vectors and the distance between their mid-points. The PDB can hence be represented by a set of labelled graphs that can be searched using a subgraph-isomorphism algorithm (as discussed here) or an MCS algorithm (as discussed in Section 8).

The precise nature of the output from a PROTEP search is determined by the tolerances that are used. The angular tolerance is specified in terms of numbers of degrees, while the distance tolerances (for the closest-approach and/or mid-point distances) are specified either in Å or as a percentage of the distance in the target structure. It is also possible to specify that the SSEs in a database protein that match the target protein are in the same sequence order as in the target; alternatively, the sequence order does not need to be the same. The user thus has a very large degree of control over the number and the quality of the matches that are identified by the program.

The use of the subgraph-isomorphism routines in PROTEP is illustrated by an extended analysis of the occurrences of β-sheet motifs in the PDB (Artymiuk et al., 1994a). Part of this study resulted in the identification of many previously-unrecognised occurrences of one particular type of β-motif, the three-stranded φ-loop (Hutchinson and Thornton, 1990). A search for a φ-loop can be executed in PROTEP by defining a pattern that consists of the angles and distances for neighbouring strands and the distance to the next-nearest neighbour strand; the Ullmann subgraph-isomorphism option is then invoked to retrieve all proteins that contain this pattern. No angular value is set for the next-nearest neighbours because of the common phenomenon of twist occurring among the strands in β-sheets, which makes it very difficult to estimate the characteristic angular values for strands other than nearest neighbours. Longer-range distances are not defined as this would impose a restraint on the overall curvature of the sheet, and the degree of twist between neighbouring strands along a sheet is seemingly unpredictable and variable from one globular protein to the next.

Such a search considers only the geometric arrangement of the strands in a β-sheet, without consideration of their sequence order. The motif's *connectivity*, *i.e.*, the form of the connections between pairs of adjacent β-strands, is determined in a second-stage search, which checks the PDB files for those structures that are retrieved by the initial PROTEP search based on geometric criteria. There are two main types of connection: in a *hairpin* connection the backbone chain re-enters the sheet on the same side as it left, whereas it re-enters on the opposite side in a *crossover* connection. In both cases the backbone loop between any two β-strands is of variable length and can take any conformation, except that it may not include another β-strand that is part of the same β-sheet. The two connected β-strands may be nearest neighbours in the β-sheet, or one or more other strands may lie between them. The connectivities are defined using the notation of Richardson (1977), where each connection is described in terms of the number of strands it moves over in the sheet and in which direction, starting from the N-terminal strand, and where an 'x is added for crossover connections. Thus, a '+1' is a hairpin and a '+1x' a crossover connection between nearest neighbour strands; a '+2' and a '+2x' are hairpin and crossover connections, respectively, that skip past one intervening strand in the β-sheet, and so on.

φ-loops are characterised by a '+2' hairpin connection between two sequentially-adjacent strands in the same β-sheet. A single φ-loop is composed of three β-strands: the two outer loops are capable of hydrogen bonding to each other but they allow the third strand to intervene between them. There are four types of φ-loop (Hutchinson and Thornton, 1990). Type 1 is the simplest φ-loop and is composed of three consecutive strands in a +2,-1 topology. A Type 1X φ-loop is characterised by a +2,-1x topology, with a crossover connection instead of the -1 hairpin. Chain reversals produce Type 1' and Type 1X' φ-loops, which are related to Types 1 and 1X and which have the topologies +1,-2 and +1x,-2, respectively. Searches for all four types of loop were carried out on the April 1992 release of the PDB, and the search results are summarised in Tables 1 and 2.

TABLE 1
Novel φ-loops identified in the Protein Data Bank (Artymiuk et al., 1994a).

Protein	Number Of φ Loops	Strand Connectivities	Residue Numbers
α-Antitrypsin (6API)	1	-1x,+2	110-195
Elongation factor TU (1ETU)	1	+2,-1	9-81
Pyrophosphatase (1PYP)	1	+2,-1	119-159
Thermolysin (7TLN)	1	+2,-1	98-124
Carboxypeptidase A (5CPA)	1	+2,-1x	47-110
	2	+2,+1x,-2	190-271
Endothiapepsin (4APE)	4	+2,+3x,-1,-1,-2	196-303
Penicillopepsin (3APP)	4	+2,+3x,-1,-1,-2	31-124
Rhizopuspepsin (3APR)	4	+2,+3x,-1,-1,-2	212-300
Pepsinogen (1PSG)	2	+2,+3x,-1,-1,-2	28-123
Glyceraldehyde-3-phosphate dehydrogenase (1GD1)	2	-2,-1,+2	169-245

Table 1 contains the φ-loops that had been identified prior to this work (Hutchinson and Thornton, 1990), while Table 2 details the new φ-loops that were discovered during this study. The simplest φ-loop (strand connectivities $+2,-1$) was found in eight distinct proteins: p21 protein catalytic domain (2P21), flavocytochrome (1FCB), chloramphenicol acetyltransferase (1CLA), cholesterol oxidase (1COX), mannose-binding protein (1MSB), fructose 1,6 biphosphate (1FBP), mesentericopeptidase (1MEE) and scorpion neurotoxin (1NRD). Type 1X loops (strand connectivities +2,-1x) were identified in proteins from four different families: isoenzyme 3-3 glutathione-5-transferase (1GST), leucine aminopeptidase (1LAP), serine carboxypeptidase (2SC2), acetylcholinesterase (1ACE). φ-loops occurring in pairs were identified in a number of members of the aspartic protease family: chymosin (2CMS), HIV protease (3HVP), Rous sarcoma virus protein (2RSP), pepsinogen (1PSG), endothiapepsin (4APE), penicillopepsin (3APP) and rhizopuspepsin (3APR), and were also identified in leucine aminopeptidase (1LAP) and purine nucleoside phosphorylase (2PNP). In all cases the pair consists of one Type 1 and one Type 1X' φ-loop and has the overall topology +2,+1x,-2. The remaining two φ-loops occur in the N-terminal regions of plastocyanin (6CPY) and pseudoazurin (2PAZ); these loops are of Type 1', which had not previously been detected in the PDB.

We have thus been able to identify a large number of previously unrecognised φ-loops, demonstrating the ability of the subgraph-isomorphism algorithm to support exploratory studies of protein structure. Further demonstrations of this ability are provided by the structural homology we have identified between the CheY bacterial signal transduction protein and EF TU, an elongation factor related to G proteins (Artymiuk *et al.*, 1990), and the resemblances that are detailed in Section 8 when discussing the MCS option in PROTEP.

5.2. Searching amino acid sidechains. The second program to be discussed here, ASSAM, has been developed for the representation and searching of patterns of amino acid sidechains in 3-D space (Artymiuk *et al.*, 1994b). The nodes in the graph representation here denote individual amino-acid sidechains and the edges denote the inter-node geometric relationships. Specifically, each node contains two *pseudo-atoms*, whose positions are chosen to emphasise the functional part of the sidechain corresponding to that node. The locations of the two pseudo-atoms are used to generate a vector, and each such vector corresponds to one of the nodes in a graph. The geometric relationships between pairs of residues are defined in terms of distances calculated between the corresponding vectors, and these relationships correspond to the edges of a graph. Specifically, if we let S, M and E denote the start, middle and end, respectively, of a vector, then the graph edges contain five parts, these being the SS, SE, ES, EE and MM distances (although only a subset of these five distances is normally used to specify a query pattern).

The vectorial representation is clearly an extremely simple description of the relative orientations of the sidechains in a 3D protein structure. It does, however, have the advantage that it does not over-define the orientations of ends of sidechains, as could occur if a more precise representation was to be used that was based directly on the individual atomic co-ordinates in the PDB. This is a useful feature for at least three reasons: in medium-resolution protein-crystallographic studies, it is often difficult to get the final torsion-angle value correct and so the fine details of the sidechain orientations may be in doubt; the identifications of the individual atoms in a residue can often be ambiguous; and sidechains can often move or twist, for example on binding substrates.

We illustrate the use of ASSAM by reference to the work of von Itzstein *et al.* (1993), who have described the design of potential anti-influenza drugs which operate by binding to a specific site on the influenza sialidase molecule, thereby inhibiting it. A key feature of the analysis was the recognition of a negatively charged patch on the sialidase surface provided by two glutamate residues and not used in the binding of sialic acid. This patch was exploited by the synthesis of a sialic acid analogue bearing an additional positive charge from either an amino-group or a guanidinyl-group appropriately placed to interact with this region of the sialidase surface.

Von Itzstein *et al.* identified a group of four sidechains as being involved in drug-binding in the influenza sialidase (two arginines, 371 and 118, and two carboxylic acid groups, glutamates 119 and 227). Co-ordinates for these sidechains were taken from the PDB sialidase structure (1NN2) and were used to generate a search pattern corresponding to this sidechain cluster. ASSAM showed that there is a very similar cluster of four sidechains in the binding pocket for the isocitrate/Mg^{2+} complex in the active site of *E. coli* isocitrate dehydrogenase (ICDH), an enzyme which catalyses the $NADP^{+}$-linked oxidative decarboxylation of isocitrate to 2-oxoglutarate.

A superimposition of the sets of sidechains from sialidase and from ICDH reveals that in ICDH the positions of arginines 119 and 153 correspond closely to the two arginines 371 and 118, respectively, in the sialidase, with excellent overlap of the guanidinium groups. In ICDH these two arginines interact with two carboxyl groups of the isocitrate, one of which, the C3 carboxyl, occupies an equivalent position to the carboxyl group of the inhibitor 4-guanidino-Neu5Ac2en in sialidase. The two carboxyl groups in the ICDH site are provided by two aspartates (aspartates 307 and 311) which are slightly displaced with respect to their counterparts in sialidase (glutamates 119 and 227 respectively). In sialidase these carboxyls co-ordinate the positive charge of the 4-guanidinyl group of the inhibitor, and in ICDH the equivalent carboxyls analogously co-ordinate the positive charge of the Mg^{2+} ion in the complex. Clearly, this result does not mean that the sialidase would necessarily be expected to bind isocitrate. The binding site for sialic acid in sialidase comprises many more residues than the two arginines and two aspartates that were highlighted by von Itzstein *et al.* and that we used as our search pattern. In fact these four residues constitute the only major area of resemblance between the binding sites in the two proteins; the folds of the polypeptide chain, and the positions of other residues in the active site, are quite different. Nevertheless, this finding does suggest that compounds with an isocitrate-like framework and a similar pattern of charge distribution might form a suitable alternative starting point for the design of new families of anti-influenza drugs.

Other structural resemblances revealed by ASSAM are discussed by Artymiuk *et al.* (1994b).

6. Identification of pharmacophoric patterns. The previous sections have demonstrated several ways in which a subgraph isomorphism algorithm can be used to search databases of chemical and biological structures. In the remainder of the paper, we consider applications of maximal common subgraph isomorphism algorithms.

Our initial studies in this area arose from work by Crandell and Smith (1983) who noted that if one had two, structurally-disparate molecules that both exhibited a biological activity of interest then, in the absence of any further information, an initial specification of the pharmacophore involved could be obtained from the MCS of the graphs representing these two molecules. Several algorithms for the identification of the MCS between pairs of 2D structures, where the MCS is defined as the largest set of (possibly connected) atoms that have matching bonds, have been described for applications such as similarity searching (Hagadone, 1992) and reaction indexing (Willett, 1986). These algorithms are, however, not suited to the processing of 3D structures, where the MCS is defined as the largest set of atoms that have matching inter-atomic distances (to within user-defined tolerance values) in the two molecules that are being compared.

The first algorithm for automatic pharmacophore identification was described by Crandell and Smith (1983). This is a breadth-first search procedure in which individual atoms common to both of the structures under investigation are systematically extended, one atom at a time, until the resulting 3D substructure cannot be extended any further. The Crandell-Smith algorithm is elegant in concept and is capable of comparing several molecules with one another, rather than just two as with many MCS algorithms. However, Brint and Willett (1987b) showed that it is very expensive, both in CPU time and in the storage space required if there is a large common substructure; in these respects, it is far inferior to MCS algorithms that are based on *clique detection* (Kuhl *et al.*, 1984; Levi, 1972).

A *clique* is a subgraph of a graph in which every node is connected to every other node and which is not contained in any larger subgraph with this property, and the MCS algorithm operates by identifying the cliques in a *correspondence graph*. Given a pair of graphs, G_1 and G_2, the correspondence graph, C, can be formed by creating the set of all pairs of nodes, one from each of the two graphs, such that the nodes of each pair are of the same type: C is then the graph whose nodes are these pairs of nodes. Two correspondence graph nodes $\{G_1(I), G_2(X)\}$ and $\{G_1(J), G_2(Y)\}$ are connected in C if the values of the edges from $G_1(I)$ to $G_1(J)$ and $G_2(X)$ to $G_2(Y)$ are the same. The maximal common subgraphs then correspond to the cliques of C, so that the identification of the MCS for a pair of 3D structures, where the nodes and edges correspond to the atoms and to the inter-atomic distances, respectively, is equivalent to the identification of the largest clique in the correspondence graph linking the two structures. Many different algorithms have been reported in the literature for clique-detection. Brint and Willett (1987b) compared the efficiencies of five of these for 3D MCS detection, and found that the algorithm of Bron and Kerbosch (1973) was by far the fastest. A worked example of the operation of this algorithm is provided by Willett (1991).

The basic Bron-Kerbosch algorithm is designed to compare just two graphs, but Brint and Willett (1987b) showed that the algorithm could be extended to find the MCS for greater numbers of 3D molecules. Their approach forms the basis for the DISCO (DIStance COmparisons) package for automatic pharmacophore detection that has been developed at Abbott Laboratories (Bures *et al.*, 1994; Martin *et al.*, 1993). DISCO identifies a bioactive conformation and superposition rule for a set of active compounds. The points for superposition are typically the ligand hydrogen-bond donor, hydrogen-bond acceptor, and charged atoms, centres of ligand hydrophobic regions, and extensions of the hydrogen bonds and electrostatic interactions to binding sites in the receptor. DISCO then uses the multi-molecule version of the clique-detection algorithm to identify the MCS for the set of input structures: the resulting *pharmacophore maps* are generated in a few minutes of CPU time. The results can be viewed in a variety of molecular modelling programs, and then used (after any appropriate modifications) as the query in a 3D pharmacophore search.

The MCS between two molecules provides an obvious measure of structural similarity, and this idea forms the basis for the 2D similarity searching system described by Hagadone (1992). It can also be used for 3D similarity searching, with the molecules in a database being ranked in decreasing order of structural overlap with the users target structure. The Bron-Kerbosch algorithm is rapid in execution but its NP-complete nature does mean that some form of screening stage is required if a rapid response is to be obtained to user queries. Upperbound procedures are appropriate when similarity, rather than substructure, searching is required (Willett, 1991) and Brint and Willett (1988) report the use of two upperbound strategies for MCS-based similarity searching. This work was partially successful in reducing the numbers of molecules that needed to undergo the time-consuming Bron-Kerbosch search, but was overtaken by later studies showing that an alternative similarity measure, called *atom mapping*, provided a more cost-effective approach to distance-based similarity searching (Pepperrell and Willett, 1991; Pepperrell *et al.*, 1990). However, we have recently described a radically different approach to similarity searching in 3D chemical databases in which the Bron-Kerbosch MCS algorithm plays a crucial role. This work is described below.

7. Matching of molecular electrostatic potentials. The small-molecule database systems that have been discussed thus far are based on the matching of atoms (or atom-like descriptors as in the pharmacophore points considered in DISCO). Such approaches take no explicit account of the electrostatic, steric and hydrophobic fields that form the basis of modern approaches to 3D QSAR (Kubinyi, 1993). An ongoing project at the University of Sheffield is hence developing methods for field-based searching, and one of the similarity searching procedures that has been developed is based on an MCS algorithm (Thorner *et al.*, 1997). The algorithm is designed to handle the molecular electrostatic potential (MEP), which has been studied previously by several groups (Burt *et al.*, 1990; Good *et al.*, 1992; Manaut *et al.* 1991; Richard, 1991), but the techniques that we have developed are applicable, in principle at least, to any field-like attribute that can be represented by real values in a 3D grid surrounding a molecule.

The electrostatic potential, P_r , at a point r for a molecule of n atoms is calculated from the point charges q_i on each atom i in the molecule, so that

$$P_r = \sum_{i=1}^{n} \frac{q_i}{|r - R_i|}$$

where R_i denotes the position of the i-th atom. A molecule is positioned at the centre of a 3D grid and the potential is calculated at each point in the grid. The similarity between a pair of molecules is estimated by aligning them so that similar features are superimposed, taking the product of the two molecular potentials at each point and then summing over the entire grid, with a suitable normalising factor being used to bring the similarities into the range -1.0 to +1.0. This numerical approach necessarily involves the matching of very large numbers of grid points and is thus extremely demanding of computational resources; however, Good *et al.* (1992) have reported an alternative approach in which the potential distribution is approximated by a series of Gaussian functions that can be processed analytically, with a substantial increase in the speed of the similarity calculation and with only a minimal effect on its accuracy. This elegant idea removes one of the main limitations of field-based approaches to 3D similarity searching, but still requires the alignment of the two molecules that are being compared prior to the calculation of the similarity, which is why field-based similarity methods have, thus far, only been applied in the context of small datasets (Vinter and Gardner, 1994).

It is simple to develop graph methods for the processing of grid-based representations of molecular fields, since a grid can be represented by a graph in which the nodes correspond to each of the grid points and in which the edges correspond to the inter-point distances. The overlap between two sets of molecular fields, and hence the similarity of the two corresponding molecules, will then be given by the overlap between the two graphs, this being estimated most obviously by their MCS. Unfortunately, existing MCS algorithms are capable of handling graphs containing only a few tens of nodes at most, whereas even a coarse molecular grid will involve many thousands of grid-points, and hence graph nodes. Accordingly, the use of an MCS algorithm for the generation of molecular alignments requires a substantial reduction in the sizes of the grid-based graphs that are to be matched, whilst ensuring that the resulting field-graphs still encompass the main features of the underlying fields so that the alignments are chemically (and hence biologically) meaningful. Once the MCS procedure has been used to generate an alignment, the similarity between the aligned molecules can be calculated using the fast Gaussian similarity procedure described previously.

A *field-graph* is generated by thresholding the grid-point values, using a user-defined threshold potential, so as to identify all the positive (or negative) grid-points with values greater (or less) than or equal to the threshold value. The resulting sub-set of the original grid-points is then considered for inclusion in one of the nodes in the field-graph, with two grid-points being allocated to the same node if they are immediately adjacent to each other. The edges of the field-graph are the distances between the centres of each of the resulting pairs of nodes, thus giving a graph that is analogous to those used for rigid 3D pharmacophore searching.

Pairs of these graphs, one representing a target structure and one representing a database structure, are matched using an MCS procedure based on the Bron-Kerbosch clique-detection algorithm. Two nodes are regarded as being equivalent if their labels have the same potential sign (either positive or negative); it is possible to adopt a more rigorous matching criterion that takes account of the magnitude of the local potential as well as its sign, or of the number of grid-points in a node, or of some combination of the two, but all our experiments have employed just the simple, sign-based matching criterion. The Bron-Kerbosch algorithm identifies the MCS based on such node-to-node matches, and the constituent pairs of matching nodes are input to a least-squares fitting routine. This routine aligns the database structure with the target structure so as to minimise the squared distances between the centroids of the field-graph nodes from the database structure and the centroids of the field-graph nodes from the target structure to which they have been mapped. The resulting alignment is then used for the final Gaussian similarity calculation.

The Bron-Kerbosch algorithm is designed, and normally used, to identify the largest subgraph common to a pair of graphs. In the present context, however, we have used it to generate all of the subgraphs common to a pair of field-graphs, and not just the largest such subgraph(s). This has been done to increase the number of possible alignments that are considered in the precise similarity calculation, and thus to ensure that the minimum possible number of close neighbours to the target structure are overlooked because of the approximations involved in the generation of the field-graphs. The similarity between an individual database structure and the target structure is taken to be the largest of the calculated similarities over all of the possible alignments resulting from the first-level, clique-detection search.

The field-graph generation procedure described above was applied to the structures in the Zeneca Agrochemicals corporate database. The 3D structures of these molecules were generated using CONCORD (Pearlman, 1987) and then the atomic point charges calculated using the MNDO routines in MOPAC Version 5.00 (Stewart, 1990). A grid was constructed around each molecule, extending for $5.0\AA$ beyond the maximum and minimum extents of the molecule in each plane, and the grids converted to field-graphs as described previously. A search of a typical target structure against the entire corporate database, containing about 173K structures, can be accomplished in about 16 hours of elapsed time on an R4000 Silicon Graphics workstation, *i.e.*, in a single overnight run, although large target structures can mean that a search will take a day or even more. Searches with the system demonstrate clearly that it often leads to the retrieval of structures with a high degree of novelty that would not be retrieved by conventional similarity searching techniques that are based on patterns of atoms (in either 2D or 3D). The system hence provides an effective way of suggesting novel bioisosteres for known active compounds. That said, the focus on just a single type of field means that while the top-ranked structures generally provide a reasonable level of MEP similarity, many of them are of little interest since their steric and/or lipophilic characteristics render them inappropriate for the biological system under investigation. The principal value of the system is hence as an ideas-generator that can suggest previously unexplored chemical classes to the chemist requesting the search, albeit at the cost (in some cases) of a low level of search precision. Further developments of this work are described by Thorner et al. (1996) and by Wild and Willett (1996).

8. Identification of common protein folding motifs. Thus far, the application of MCS algorithms to the 3D protein structures in the PDB has been at the levels of the SSEs, using the representation of the α-helix and β-strand elements that has been discussed in Section 5.1 and using the Bron-Kerbosch algorithm to identify the MCS. In fact, the algorithm has been implemented so that it will retrieve all of the proteins in the PDB that contain at least some minimum number of the SSEs in the query pattern (which is thus normally an entire structure, rather than a partial structure as is the case when the Ullmann option in PROTEP is used). This has been one of the most productive applications of graph theory that we have identified thus far, as demonstrated by the structural resemblances that we have discovered and that are listed in Table 3. Here, we discuss two of these resemblances.

The first example is a previously unknown resemblance between three otherwise-unrelated proteins: prealbumin (2PAB), protocatechuate 3,4-dioxygenase (1PCD) and thaumatin (1THI) (Artymiuk *et al.*, 1995). A search using 1PCD as the target structure showed that it shared a common β-sandwich fold with the other two proteins: the common fold consisted of one three-stranded and one four-stranded β-sheet, these motifs comprising a major part of the mixed β-sandwich found in each protein.

Human prealbumin (which is also known as transthyretin) is a hormone binding protein which has two thyroxine-binding sites and also independent binding sites for retinol binding protein, the specific plasma carrier of vitamin A. The crystal structure has been solved to $1.8\AA$ resolution and detailed binding studies have revealed the nature of the substrate specificity sites. The molecule is a tetramer of identical subunits, each containing 127 amino acid residues and consisting of an 8-stranded β-barrel structure organised into two 4-stranded β-sheets, together with a short stretch of α-helix. Protocatechuate $3,4$-dioxygenase belongs to a family of bacterial

TABLE 2
Previously unrecognised structural resemblances identified by use of a maximal common subgraph isomorphism algorithm.

Protein	Number of φ Loops	Strand Connectivities	Residue Number
Plastocyanin (6PCY)	1	+1,-2	1-32
Pseudoazurin (2PAZ)	1	+1,-2	1-35
Chloramphenicol acetyltransferase (1CLA)	1	-1,+2	89-151
Flavocytochrome (1FCB)	1	-1,+2	25-85
Fructose 1,6 biphosphate (1FBP)	1	-1,+2	93-115
Scorpion neurotoxin (1NRD)	1	-1,+2	263-296
Isoenzyme 3-3 glutathione-5-transferase (1GST)	1	-1x,+2	2-64
Cholesterol oxidase (1COX)	1	+2,-1	283-473
Mannose-binding protein (1MSB)	1	+2,-1	180-208
Mesentericopeptidase (1MEE)	1	+2,-1	197-268
P21 protein catalytic domain (2P21)	1	+2,-1	1-58
Acetylcholinesterase (1ACE)	1	+2,-1x	95-147
Carboxypeptidase A (5CPA)	1	+2,-1x	47-110
Leucine aminopeptidase (1LAP)	1	+2,-1x	227-301
	2	+2,+1x,-2	352-450
Serine carboxypeptidase (2SC2)	1	+2,-1x	31-95
Chymosin (2CMS)	2	+2,+1x,-2	31-126
Endothiapepsin (4APE)	2	+2,+1x,-2	29-123
Pepsinogen (1PSG)	2	+2,+1x,-2	209-303
Penicillopepsin (3APP)	2	+2,+1x,-2	208-299
Rhizopuspepsin (3APR)	2	+2,+1x,-2	30-125
Purine nucleoside phosphorylase (2PNP)	2	+2,+1x,-2	110-241
HIV proteinase (3HVP)	2	+2,+3x,-1,-1,-2	22-79
Rous sarcoma virus protein (2RSP)	2	+2,+3x,-1,-1,-2	34-110

dioxygenases that catalyse the cleavage of molecular oxygen with the subsequent incorporation of both oxygen atoms into organic substrates. The molecule is an oligomer of dissimilar subunits, the α-subunit containing 200 residues and the β-subunit containing 238 residues. Both subunits share a common structural core, which consists of a flattened 9-stranded β-barrel and three short α-helices, but they differ in their terminii and in several surface loops. Thaumatin is a monomeric (207 residues), intensely sweet protein of unknown function, which is extracted from the fruit of an African plant *Thaumatococcus danielli*. The crystal structure has been solved at 3.0Å resolution and reveals a flattened 11-stranded β-barrel, surrounded by many loops closed by disulphide bonds.

The 3D resemblance in the common region is good, with the RMSD over the equivalenced residues ranging from 0.91 (for the three-stranded motif in 2PAB and 1PCD) to 2.35Å (for the four-stranded motif in 1THI and 1PCD). The superpositions show an identical organisation and order of the strands, which also appear to be conserved in position, although the four-stranded motif in 1THI/1PCD superposed less well than the others. A detailed multiple-alignment study failed to identify any statistically-significant sequence homologies between the residues comprising the common structural feature in the three proteins and the question then arises as to why there is such a strong structural resemblance despite the lack of any sequence resemblance. Three possible explanations suggest themselves.

Firstly, it is possible that the proteins may be evolutionarily related, but so remotely that all significant sequence homology has been lost, and only a common substructure remains. An alternative possibility is that some members of the three families may bind to structurally-similar receptors. This explanation could arise by evolutionary processes, and would thus be compatible with the previous suggestion. However, the three proteins are extremely diverse and are not known to bind structurally-similar receptors. Thus, in this case, there seems no reason to believe that there could be any evolutionary similarity; accordingly, the previous explanations are unlikely and we instead believe that the observed 3D resemblance simply reflects a particularly stable folding motif. Two pieces of evidence support this suggestion. First, the common fold between 2PAB, 1PCD and 1THI resembles the β-sandwich found in azurin (1AZA), another unrelated protein. Second, five of the β-strands in the common fold between 2PAB, 1PCD and 1THI are structurally very similar to five of the β-strands in a Type 1 jelly role, a stable structural feature that is found in a wide variety of unrelated molecules (Gibson and Argos, 1990). Consequently, it is quite possible that the common fold identified in this work is simply a modification of a particularly stable folding motif, rather than an example of an evolutionary relationship (Artymiuk *et al.*, 1995).

An evolutionary relationship is much more likely in the second example to be discussed here (Artymiuk *et al.*, 1996), which involves biotin carboxylase (BC) and the family of ADP-forming peptide synthetases, as represented by D-alanine:D-alanine ligase (DD-ligase) and glutathione reductase (GSHase). Fan *et al.* (1995) have reported the existence of a strong similarity between the structures of DD-ligase, a bacterial cell-wall synthesising enzyme, and GSHase. Both proteins consist of three domains with similar folds, and both convert ATP to ADP as part of a ligation reaction which leads to the creation of a peptide bond. Although there is very little sequence homology between the two proteins, the 3D similarities are so strong that Fan *et al.* argued for an evolutionary relationship between the two enzymes, and postulated that their common structure may represent a general fold for that class of peptide synthetases that cleave ATP to ADP, rather than to AMP.

PROTEP was able to demonstrate a further striking similarity between the folds of GSHase and DD-ligase and that of BC. The similarities are so extensive as to be strongly suggestive of an evolutionary relationship between BC and the peptide ligases, showing that this family of protein structures is much wider than previously suspected and extends beyond the peptide synthetases to the large family of biotin-dependent carboxylases.

The similarity between BC and GSHase and DD-ligase is wide-ranging and involves a total of nine α-helices and 13 β-strands, all with identical sequence and topology. The resemblance involves virtually all of the GSHase and DD-ligase folds with the first 318 residues of the BC fold. Overall, the folds are exceedingly similar, although there are minor differences in the arrangement of the β-strands at the periphery of the N-terminal β-sheet in all three enzymes. Between BC and GSHase it is possible to superpose 101 Cα atoms with an RMSD of 1.91Å; the similarity between BC and DD-ligase is even greater with 127 Cα atoms superposing with an RMSD of 1.64Å.

The similarities extend to the positions of the active sites of the three enzymes, although the assignment is rather tentative for BC because of difficulties in carrying out binding studies in the crystalline state. Moreover, there are also significant resemblances when the functional and mechanistic characteristics of the three enzymes are examined. The reactions they catalyse are similar, coupling the conversion of ATP to ADP to form a carbon-nitrogen bond between a carboxyl group and an amino group: BC ligates ATP-activated bicarbonate to the N1' amino group of biotin to produce carboxy-biotin; GSHase ligates the ATP-activated carboxyl of γ-Glu-Cys to the amino group of glycine to produce glutathione; and DD-ligase ligates the ATP-activated carboxyl group of D-alanine to the amino group of another D-alanine. The differences in chemistry relate to the fact that in BC the reaction catalysed involves a secondary amine, whilst in GSHase and DD-ligase, the reaction involves a primary amine. However, despite this difference, the mechanisms of both classes of enzyme appear to be similar: the GSHase and DD-ligase reactions proceed through acylphosphate intermediaries, and it is believed that the reaction catalysed by BC proceeds through the analogous carboxyphosphate intermediate. Given these structural and mechanistic resemblances, it is not unreasonable to postulate the existence of a common evolutionary ancestor between BC and GSHase and DD-ligase, and this is supported by detailed homology studies that reveal several areas of significant sequence similarity within the three enzymes.

BC is a member of a large family of homologous ADP-forming biotin-dependent carboxylases which includes carbamoyl-phosphate synthetase, proprionyl-CoA carboxylase, pyruvate carboxylase and L-glutamine-amido-ligase, and the study reported here hence unites this family of enzymes with the family of ADP-forming peptide synthetases (as represented by DD-ligase and GSHase) (Artymiuk *et al.*, 1996).

TABLE 3

φ-loops in the Protein Data Bank identified by Hutchinson and Thornton (1990).

Related Proteins	Common Features	Comments
Leucine aminopeptidase and carboxypeptidase	Eight β-strands in a sheet plus five α-helices	Minimal sequence homology even in the area of structural overlap
Ribonuclease H domain of HIV-1 reverse transcriptase (RT) and the ATPase folds of hexokinase, heat-shock cognate protein and actin	Five β-strands in a sheet plus one α-helix.	No other proteins in the PDB contain this β-sheet. The common motif also occurs in an intramolecular resemblance between the same ribonuclease *H* domain of RT and two other domains of RT
Prealbumin, protocatechuate 3,4-dioxygenase and thaumatin	One three-stranded and one four-stranded β-sheet.	Resemblance probably due to a particularly stable folding motif
Biotin synthetic/repressor protein and serine tRNA	Seven β-strands, with two α-helices on either side of the sheet	No other proteins in the PDB contain this β-motif
β-Glucosyltransferase and glycogen phosphorylase	13 β-strands and eight α-helices, plus a further two strands and three helices additional to the large core feature	Structural and chemical similarities suggest a remote evolutionary relationship.
Enoyl ACP reductase and $3\alpha, 20\beta$-hydroxysteroid dehydrogenase	Seven β-strands and four α-helices	Possible evolutionary relationship
D-alanine:D-alanine ligase, glutathione reductase and biotin carboxylase	13 β-strands and nine α-helices	Structural and mechanistic similarities provide strong evidence for an evolutionary relationship.

9. Conclusions. In this paper, we have provided an overview of the work carried out in the University of Sheffield over the last few years into the use of isomorphism algorithms for searching databases of chemical and biological structures. We have shown that the subgraph and MCS isomorphism algorithms that have been used previously for searching 2D small molecules can also be used for: substructure searching in the Complex Carbohydrate Sequence Database (CCSD); for 3D substructure searching in both small molecules and proteins; for pharmacophore mapping; for field-based similarity searching; and for the analysis of protein folding motifs.

The emphasis of the paper has been on the applications, rather than on the detailed implementation of the various graph-based procedures we have developed. However, while it is important that the procedures are effective, their use in a database context requires that they also be efficient, and several of our studies have thus involved detailed comparisons of the efficiencies of published subgraph or MCS algorithms to ascertain their suitability for processing chemical and biological databases (Brint and Willett, 1987a, 1987b; Downs *et al.*, 1988; Willett, 1991). These studies have demonstrated the general utility of the Ullmann and Bron-Kerbosch algorithms, and we have been heartened by the extent to which others have taken them up for use in a wide range of chemical and biological applications (see, e.g., Martin *et al.*, 1993; Sheridan *et al.*, 1989). It is, however, the case that new algorithms continue to appear in the literatures of subjects such as computer science, graph theory and operations research (see, e.g., Pardalos and Xue, 1994); we consequently try to maintain a "watching brief" on this literature to see if it is possible to identify new algorithms that are still more efficient than those that form the current bases of our various programs.

It is most important that graph matching algorithms are tested using data with characteristics typical of the application domain in which they are to be used. Algorithmic testing normally involves either random graphs, or graphs that have been deliberately designed to be as complex, and thus difficult to solve, as possible: such graphs are unlikely to bear much resemblance to those used for the representation of chemical and biological molecules. For example, Gardiner (1996) has recently compared a new clique-detection algorithm due to Babel (1991) with the Bron-Kerbosch algorithm. This branch-and-bound algorithm is straightforward in concept and has been shown to out-perform all existing algorithms when used for clique-detection in random graphs containing up to 1,000 nodes. Unfortunately, when tested with pairs of 3D small molecules, the algorithm was found to be faster than the Bron-Kerbosch algorithm only when processing graphs having a high *edge density*, a parameter that describes the probability that two nodes in the correspondence graph will be linked in the largest clique. This will occur either if the two molecules that are being compared have an extremely large MCS (in which case the resemblances are likely to be obvious) or if very large matching tolerances are employed (in which case it is possible to obtain large MCSs even with molecules having little or no relationship with each other). Accordingly, while the Babel algorithm can process random graphs extremely rapidly, it does not appear to be appropriate for the applications considered here.

In conclusion, we wish to emphasise that, despite the many successful applications we have described, it should not be assumed that *any* sort of structure-matching application may be implemented using graph isomorphism methods. Firstly, we have already noted that both subgraph and maximal common subgraph isomorphism are NP-complete problems, and thus extremely demanding of computational resources unless effective procedures are available for minimising the number of node-to-node comparisons required for the matching of a pair of structures. Fortunately, this is the case with the graphs representing chemical or biological molecules, where fast matching is possible because of the discriminating labels associated with each of the nodes and edges, *e.g.*, elemental types and interatomic distances in the case of the graph representing a 3D small molecule. Even with this wealth of information, run-times can become very long if the graphs that are to be matched contain very large numbers of nodes; indeed, storage can also become a problem for MCS-based applications, since clique-detection has a storage complexity of $O(N^4)$ for graphs containing N nodes. Secondly, while graph-based procedures are well suited to matching individual conformations of flexible molecules, alternative computational paradigms may be necessary if there is a need to explore torsional space fully, as is increasingly the case when seeking to identify novel bioactive molecules (Martin and Willett, 1997). In such cases, one may be forced to use non-deterministic approaches that may result in sub-optimal solutions but that do at least enable a solution to be achieved, whereas this might well not be possible with graph-based methods. There has accordingly been much interest in the use of non-deterministic approaches - such as simulated annealing, neural networks and genetic algorithms - for matching chemical and biological structures. For example, we are making increasing use of genetic algorithms for applications such as MCS-identification when very large 2D chemical graphs need to be processed (Brown *et al.*, 1994) and for pharmacophore mapping (Jones *et al.*, 1995) and field-based similarity searching (Thorner *et al.*, 1996) when flexible, rather than rigid, 3D structures need to be processed. Even so, we believe that graph theoretic approaches will continue to play an important role in the development of new methods for accessing the increasing amounts of structural information in chemical and biological databases.

Acknowledgements. It is a pleasure to acknowledge the contributions of the following individuals to the work that has been carried out in my group on chemical and biological applications of graph theory: Peter Artymiuk, Andrew Brint, Ian Bruno, David Clark, Geoff Downs, Eleanor

Gardiner, Helen Grindley, Susan Jakes, Nick Kemp, Andrew Poirrette, Eleanor Mitchell, David Rice, David Thorner, Elizabeth Ujah and Matt Wright. Funding for these studies has been provided by: the Biotechnology and Biological Sciences Research Council, the British Library Research and Development Department, the Cambridge Crystallographic Data Centre, the James Black Foundation, the Medical Research Council, Pfizer Central Research, the Science and Engineering Research Council, Tripos Inc., Zeneca Agrochemicals and Zeneca Pharmaceuticals. The Krebs Institute for Biomolecular Research is a designated Biomolecular Sciences Centre of the Biotechnology and Biological Sciences Research Council.

REFERENCES

Artymiuk, P. J., Grindley, H. M., MacKenzie, A. B., Rice, D. W., Ujah, E. C. and Willett, P. (1995). PROTEP: a program for graph-theoretic similarity searching of the 3-D structures in the Protein Data Bank. In: Carbo, R. (editor) *Molecular Similarity and Reactivity: from Quantum Chemical to Phenomenological Approaches*. Netherlands: Kluwer Academic Publishers.

Artymiuk, P. J., Grindley, H. M., Poirrette, A. R., Rice, D. W., Ujah, E. C. and Willett, P. (1994a). Identification of β-sheet motifs, of φ-loops, and of patterns of amino-acid residues in three-dimensional protein structures using a subgraph-isomorphism algorithm. *Journal of Chemical Information and Computer Sciences*, 34, 54–62.

Artymiuk, P. J., Poirrette, A. R., Grindley, H. M., Rice, D. W. and Willett, P. (1994b). A graph-theoretic approach to the identification of three-dimensional patterns of amino acid sidechains in protein structures. *Journal of Molecular Biology*, 243, 327–344.

Artymiuk, P. J., Poirrette, A. R., Rice, D. W. and Willett, P. (1996). Biotin carboxylase comes into the fold. *Nature Structural Biology*, 3, 128–132.

Artymiuk, P. J., Rice, D. W., Mitchell, E. M. and Willett, P. (1990). Structural resemblance between the families of bacterial signal-transduction proteins and of *G* proteins revealed by graph theoretical techniques. *Protein Engineering*, 4, 39–43.

Ash, J. E., Warr, W. A. and Willett, P. (editors) (1991). *Chemical Structure Systems*. Chichester: Ellis Horwood.

Babel, L. (1991). Finding maximum cliques in arbitray and special graphs. *Computing*, 46, 321–341.

Barnard, J. M. (1993). Substructure searching methods: old and new. *Journal of Chemical Information and Computer Sciences*, 33, 532–538.

Bernstein, F. C., Koetzle, T. F., Williams, G. J. B., Meyer, E. F. Jnr., Brice, M. D., Rodgers, J. R., Kennard, O., Shimanouchi, M. and Tasumi, M. (1977). The Protein Data Bank: a computer-based archival file for macromolecular structures. *Journal of Molecular Biology*, 112, 535–542.

Brint, A. T. and Willett, P. (1987a). Pharmacophoric pattern matching in files of 3-D chemical structures: comparison of geometric searching algorithms. *Journal of Molecular Graphics*, 5, 49–56.

Brint, A. T. and Willett, P. (1987b). Algorithms for the identification of three-dimensional maximal common substructures. *Journal of Chemical Information and Computer Sciences*, 27, 152–158.

Brint, A. T. and Willett, P. (1988). Upperbound procedures for the identification of similar three-dimensional chemical structures. *Journal of Computer-Aided Molecular Design*, 2, 311–320.

Bron, C. and Kerbosch, J. (1973). Algorithm 457. Finding all cliques of an undirected graph. *Communications of the ACM*, 16, 575–577.

Brown, R. D., Jones, G., Willett, P. and Glen, R. C. (1994). Matching two-dimensional chemical graphs using genetic algorithms. *Journal of Chemical Information and*

Computer Sciences, 34, 63–70.

Bruno, I. J., Kemp, N. M., Artymiuk, P. J. and Willett, P. (1997). Representation and searching of carbohydrate structures using graph-theoretic techniques, submitted for publication.

Bures, M. G. (1997) Intergration of molecular modelling and database searching. In: Martin, Y. C. and Willett, P. (editors) (1997) *Designing Bioactive Molecules: Three-Dimensional Techniques and Applications*. Washington DC: American Chemical Society, in the press.

Bures, M. G., Danaher, E., DeLazzer, J. and Martin, Y. C. (1994). New molecular modelling tools using three-dimensional chemical substructures. *Journal of Chemical Information and Computer Sciences*, 34, 218–223.

Burt, C., Richards, W. H. and Huxley, P. (1990). The application of molecular similarity calculations. *Journal of Computational Chemistry*, 11, 1139–1146.

Clark, D. E., Jones, G., Willett, P., Kenny, P. W. and Glen, R. C. (1994). Pharmacophoric pattern matching in files of three-dimensional chemical structures: comparison of conformational-searching algorithms for flexible searching. *Journal of Chemical Information and Computer Sciences*, 34, 197–206.

Clark, D. E., Willett, P. and Kenny, P. W. (1992). Pharmacophoric pattern matching in files of three-dimensional chemical structures: use of smoothed bounded-distance matrices for the representation and searching of conformationally-flexible molecules. *Journal of Molecular Graphics*, 10, 194–204.

Crandell, C. W. and Smith, D. H. (1983). Computer-assisted examination of compounds for common three-dimensional substructures. *Journal of Chemical Information and Computer Sciences*, 23, 186–197.

Cringean, J. K., Pepperrell, C. A., Poirrette, A. R. and Willett, P. (1990). Selection of screens for three-dimensional substructure searching. *Tetrahedron Computer Methodology*, 3, 37–46.

Crippen, G. M. and Havel, T. F. (1988). *Distance Geometry and Molecular Conformation*. Letchworth: Research Studies Press.

Doubet, S., Bock, K., Smith, D., Darvill, A. and Albersheim, P. (1989). The Complex Carbohydrate Structure Database. *Trends in Biochemical Sciences*, 14, 475–477.

Downs, G. M., Lynch, M. F., Willett, P., Manson, G. A. and Wilson, G. A. (1988). Transputer implementations of chemical substructure searching algorithms. *Tetrahedron Computer Methodology*, 1, 207–217.

Downs, G. M. and Willett, P. (1996) Similarity searching in databases of chemical structures. *Reviews in Computational Chemistry*, 7, 1–66.

Fan, C., Moews, P. C., Shi, Y., Walsh, C. T. and Knox, J. R. (1995). A common fold for peptide synthetases cleaving ATP to ADP – glutathione synthetase and D-Alanine-D-Alanine ligase of *Escherichia Coli*. *Proceedings of the National Academy of Sciences of the USA*, 92, 1172–1176.

Feizi, T. and Bundle, D. (1996) Carbohydrates and glycoconjugates. The coming age for oligosaccharide ligands and databases for saccharide structures. słCurrent Opinion in Structural Biology, 6, 659–662.

Fisanick, W., Cross, K. P. and Rusinko, A. (1992). Similarity searching on CAS Registry substances. 1. Global molecular property and generic atom triangle geometric searching. *Journal of Chemical Information and Computer Sciences*, 32, 664–674.

Gardiner, E. (1996) *An Evaluation of a New Clique-Detection Procedure for Matching Chemical Structures*. MSc dissertation, University of Sheffield.

Garey, M. R. and Johnson, D. S. (1979). *Computers and Intractability: a Guide to the Theory of NP-Completeness*. San Francisco: W. H. Freeman.

Gati, G. (1979). Further annotated bibliography on the isomorphism disease. *Journal of Graph Theory*, 3, 95–109.

Gibson, T. J. and Argos, P. (1990). Protruding domain of tomato bushy stunt virus coat protein is a hitherto unrecognized class of jellyroll conformation. *Journal of Molecular Biology*, 212, 7–9.

Good, A. C., Hodgkin, E. E. and Richards, W. G. (1992). The utilisation of Gaussian functions for the rapid evaluation of molecular similarity. *Journal of Chemical Information and Computer Science*, 32, 188–191.

Good, A. C. and Mason, J. S. (1996). Three-dimensional structure database searches. Reviews in *Computational Chemistry*, 7, 67–117.

Gund, P. (1977). Three-dimensional pharmacophoric pattern searching. *Progress in Molecular and Subcellular Biology*, 5, 117–143.

Hagadone, T. R. (1992). Molecular subsimilarity searching: efficient retrieval in two-dimensional structure databases. *Journal of Chemical Information and Computer Sciences*, 32, 515–521.

Hodes, L. (1976). Selection of descriptors according to discrimination and redundancy. Application to chemical substructure searching. *Journal of Chemical Information and Computer Sciences*, 16, 88–93.

Hurst, T. (1994). Flexible 3D searching: the directed tweak technique. *Journal of Chemical Information and Computer Sciences*, 34, 190–196.

Hutchinson, E. G. and Thornton, J. M. (1990). HERA – A program to draw schematic diagrams of protein secondary structures. *Proteins: Structure, Function, and Genetics*, 8, 203–212.

Jakes, S. E. and Willett, P. (1986). Pharmacophoric pattern matching in files of 3-D chemical structures: selection of inter-atomic distance screens. *Journal of Molecular Graphics*, 4, 12–20.

Jones, G., Willett, P. and Glen, R. C. (1995). A genetic algorithm for flexible molecular overlay and pharmacophore detection. *Journal of Computer-Aided Molecular Design*, 9, 532–549.

Kubinyi, H. (1993) (editor). *3D QSAR in Drug Design*. Leiden: ESCOM.

Kuhl, F. S., Crippen, G. M. and Friesen, D. K. (1984). A combinatorial algorithm for calculating ligand binding. *Journal of Computational Chemistry*, 5, 24–34.

Leach, A. R. (1991). A survey of methods for searching the conformational space of small and medium-sized molecules. *Reviews in Computational Chemistry*, 2, 1–55.

Levi, G. (1972). A note on the derivation of maximal common subgraphs of two directed or undirected graphs. *Calcolo*, 9, 341–352.

McGregor, J. J. (1982). Backtrack search algorithms and the maximal common subgraph problem. *Software Practice and Experience*, 12, 23–34.

Manaut, F., Sanz, F., Jose, J. and Milesi, M. (1991). Automatic search for maximum similarity between molecular electrostatic potential distributions. *Journal of Computer-Aided Molecular Design*, 5, 371–380.

Martin, Y. C., Bures, M. G., Danaher, E. A., DeLazzer, J., Lico, I. and Pavlik, P. A. (1993). A fast new approach to pharmacophore mapping and its application to dopaminergic and benzodiazepine agonists. *Journal of Computer-Aided Molecular Design*, 7, 83–102.

Martin, Y. C. and Willett, P. (editors) (1997) *Designing Bioactive Molecules: Three-Dimensional Techniques and Applications*. Washington DC: American Chemical Society, in the press.

Mitchell, E. M., Artymiuk, P. J., Rice, D. W. and Willett, P. (1990). Use of techniques derived from graph theory to compare secondary structure motifs in proteins. *Journal of Molecular Biology*, 212, 151–166.

Morgan, H. L. (1965). The generation of a unique machine description for chemical structures: a technique developed at Chemical Abstracts Service. *Journal of Chemical Documentation*, 5, 107–113.

Nilakantan, R., Bauman, N. and Venkataraghavan, R. (1993). A new method for rapid characterisation of molecular shape: applications in drug design. *Journal of Chemical Information and Computer Sciences*, 33, 79–85.

Pardalos, P. M. and Xue, J. (1994). The maximum clique problem. *Journal of Global Optimization*, 4, 301–328.

Pearlman, R. S. (1987). Rapid generation of high quality approximate 3D molecular structures. *Chemical Design Automation News*, 2, 1–6.

Pepperrell, C. A. and Willett, P. (1991). Techniques for the calculation of three-

dimensional structural similarity using inter-atomic distances. *Journal of Computer-Aided Molecular Design*, 5, 455–474.
Pepperrell, C. A., Willett, P. and Taylor, R. (1990). Implementation and use of an atom-mapping procedure for similarity searching in databases of 3-D chemical structures. *Tetrahedron Computer Methodology*, 3, 575–593.
Poirrette, A. R., Willett, P. and Allen, F. H. (1991). Pharmacophoric pattern matching in files of three-dimensional chemical structures: characterisation and use of generalised valence angle screens. *Journal of Molecular Graphics*, 9, 203–217.
Poirrette, A. R., Willett, P. and Allen, F. H. (1993). Pharmacophoric pattern matching in files of three-dimensional chemical structures: characterisation and use of generalised torsion angle screens. *Journal of Molecular Graphics*, 11, 2–14.
Ray, L. C. and Kirsch, R. A. (1957). Finding chemical records by digital computers. *Science*, 126, 814–819.
Read, R. C. and Corneil, D. G. (1977). The graph isomorphism disease. *Journal of Graph Theory*, 1, 339–363.
Richard, A. M. (1991). Quantitative comparison of molecular electrostatic potentials for structure-activity studies. *Journal of Computational Chemistry*, 12, 959–969.
Richardson, J. S. (1977). β-sheet topology and the relatedness of proteins. Nature, 268, 495–500.
Sadowski, J. and Gasteiger, J. (1993). From atoms and bonds to three-dimensional atomic coordinates: automatic model builders. *Chemical Reviews*, 93, 2567–2581.
Sheridan, R. P., Nilakantan, R., Rusinko, A., Bauman, N., Haraki, K. S. and Venkataraghavan, R. (1989). 3DSEARCH: a system for three-dimensional substructure searching. *Journal of Chemical Information and Computer Sciences*, 29, 255–260.
Stewart, J. J. M. (1990). MOPAC: a semi-empirical molecular orbital program. *Journal of Computer-Aided Molecular Design*, 4, 1–105.
Sussenguth, E. H. (1965). A graph-theoretic algorithm for matching chemical structures. *Journal of Chemical Documentation*, 5, 36–43.
Thorner, D. A., Willett, P., Wright, P. M. and Taylor, R. (1997). Similarity searching in files of three-dimensional chemical structures: representation and searching of molecular electrostatic potentials using field-graphs. *Journal of Computer-Aided Molecular Design*, 11, 163–174.
Thorner, D. A., Wild, D. J, Willett, P. and Wright, P. M. (1996). Similarity searching in files of three-dimensional chemical structures: flexible field-based searching of molecular electrostatic potentials. *Journal of Chemical Information and Computer Sciences*, 36, 900–908.
Trinajstic, N. (editor) (1983). *Chemical Graph Theory*. Chichester: Ellis Horwood.
Ullmann, J. R. (1976). An algorithm for subgraph isomorphism. *Journal of the Association for Computing Machinery*, 23, 31–42.
Vinter, J. G. and Gardner, M. (editors) (1994). *Molecular Modelling and Drug Design*. London: Macmillan.
von Itzstein, M., Wu, W.-Y., Kok, G. B., Pegg, M. S., Dyason, J. C., Jin, B., Phan, T. V., Smythe, M. L., White, H. F., Oliver, S. W., Colman, P. M., Varghese, J. N., Ryan, D. M., Woods, J. M., Bethell, R. C., Hotham, V. J., Cameron, J. M. and Penn, C. R. (1993). Rational design of potent sialidase-based inhibitors of influenza-virus replication. *Nature*, 363, 418–423.
Warr, W. A. and Willett, P. (1997). The principles and practice of 3D database searching. In: Martin, Y. C. and Willett, P. (editors) *Designing Bioactive Molecules: Three-Dimensional Techniques and Applications*. Washington DC: American Chemical Society, in the press.
Wild, D. J and Willett, P. (1996). Similarity searching in files of three-dimensional chemical structures: alignment of Molecular Electrostatic Potentials with a genetic algorithm. *Journal of Chemical Information and Computer Sciences*, 36, 159–167.
Willett, P. (editor) (1986). *Modern Approaches to Chemical Reaction Searching*. Aldershot: Gower.
Willett, P. (1991). *Three-Dimensional Chemical Structure Handling*. Taunton: Research Studies Press.
Wilson, R. (1972). *Introduction to Graph Theory*. Edinburgh: Oliver and Boyd.

MOLECULAR SIMILARITY

W. GRAHAM RICHARDS* AND DANIEL D. ROBINSON†

Abstract. Molecular similarity aims to give a quantitative answer to the question of how similar two given molecules are. Such indices are of use in drug design as aids to the creation of molecular mimics and in structure- activity studies or measures of molecular diversity. Similarity is most often computed in terms of molecular shape or electrostatic potential.

The advent of combinatorial techniques and the use of high throughput synthesis have created a need for ever faster methods of computation. Numerical calculation has been superceded by analytical evaluation of integrals, but even faster methods are urgently needed. This is especially so if we can ever hope to take thousands of molecules and calculate the similarity between all pairs.

A promising technique is to use two-dimensional molecular representations and to utilise methodologies perfected in optical character recognition.

1. Introduction. Molecular similarity aims to give a simple quantitative answer to the question, "How similar is molecule A to molecule B?"

If we can provide a single number which is a measure of similarity it will have a range of useful applications.

1. Similarity helps in the design of mimetics or bioisoteres.
2. The vexed problem of optimally aligning molecules in order to make comparisons may be alleviated.
3. Similarities between all pairs of a set of compounds may provide the basis for structure-activity correlations in respect of pharmacological activity.
4. Similarity provides a measure of diversity.

What is needed is a simple numerical index of similarity, and a number of such measures have been proposed.

In this short paper we are not attempting to present an extensive review of molecular similarity so that there are no references to the many variations on the idea. Rather we are focussing on the problems presented by the need for speed in such calculations. One major problem, that of how to deal with conformationally flexible molecules, we likewise bypass with the result that for such species we will be calculating similarity for selected conformations and not selecting conformers. We also concentrate on the similarity between entire ungelded molecules, although we could in principle apply the techniques to parts of molecules or pharmacophores

2. Similarity indices. We imagine having two three-dimensional molecules, A and B, superimposed and then compute some property ρ_A of

*New Chemistry Laboratory, Oxford University, South Parks Road, Oxford OX1 3QT, United Kingdom.

† Department of Chemistry, Oxford University, South Parks Road, Oxford OX1 3QZ, United Kingdom.

A and ρ_B of B at points in space surrounding the molecules. A formula due to Carbo [1] expresses similarity as:

$$\text{Similarity} = \frac{\int \rho_A \rho_B d\tau}{\sqrt{\int \rho_A^2 d\tau \int \rho_B^2 d\tau}}$$

that is an overlap of the properties divided by a normalizing denominator which constrains the value to the range zero to one.

This formula is by no means unique, for example an alternative due to Hodgkin and the author [2] takes the form:

$$\text{Similarity} = \frac{2\int \rho_A \rho_B d\tau}{\int \rho_A^2 d\tau + \int \rho_B^2 d\tau}$$

The latter formalism avoids a possible problem when $\rho_A = n\rho_B$, where the first formula would indicate identity, but in practice there appears to be no strong reason for preferring one form over the other. Some recent work also suggests that there may be some advantage in not including the normalization. This certainly improves the speed of the calculation which as we shall see is an important factor.

The early uses of similarity employed electron density obtained from quantum mechanical wavefunctions as the property ρ, and replaced integration by summation over a coarse three dimensional grid.

The context of much of the use of similarity has been in drug design where the molecular scenario envisaged is that of a small molecule binding to a specific site on a macromolecule. The all important binding energy will be a combination of attractive forces and repulsion. Thus, rather than using electron density as the property relative to which similarity is judged, quantities more obviously related to intermolecular forces are preferred.

For attraction an obvious and much utilised choice is the molecular electrostatic potential: the value at a given point is the interaction energy of an isolated proton at that position. This property has the advantage of being more discriminating, since it can take both positive and negative values. Alternatively the derivative of the electrostatic field might offer some useful qualities. Generally again little difference is observed in practice although one might envisage that electrostatic potential would be more appropriate for ionic interactions and the field for dipolar bonding.

In both the case of potential and that of field, the value will vary as an inverse power of the distance of the point of calculation from atomic nuclei. Hence if we are using numerical methods and a grid point coincides with a nuclear position, then the value of the property will become infinite. The simple way of avoiding such an anomaly is to compute the values of the property only in the regions of space outside the van der Waals envelope of the molecules.

A better way of avoiding this latter complexity is to perform the necessary integrals analytically rather than numerically. That may be achieved by fitting the form $1/r$ to a trio of Gaussian functions and performing the integrals using the code developed for calculating Gaussian integrals [3]. Putting this more formally, we may evaluate the electrostatic potential at a given point r in a molecule of N atoms, each with a point charge q_i as:

$$p_r = \sum_{i=1}^{N} \frac{q_i}{(r - R_i)}$$

where R_i is the nuclear coordinate position of atom i. It is possible to substitute the $1/r$ term in the above equation with a Gaussian function approximation:

$$p_r = \sum_{i=1}^{N} q_i(\gamma_1 e^{-\alpha_1(r-R_i)^2} + \gamma_2 e^{-\alpha_2(r-R_i)^2} + ...\gamma_k e^{-\alpha_k(r-R_i)^2})$$

If this equation is inserted into the Carbo formula we get the following equation:

Similarity=

$$\frac{\left[\sum_{i=1}^{N}\sum_{j=1}^{M} q_i q_j \int (G_1^i+G_2^i+...G_k^i)\times(G_1^j+G_2^j+...G_k^j)d\tau\right]}{\sqrt{\left[\sum_{i=1}^{N}\sum_{i=1}^{N} q_i q_i \int (G_1^i+G_2^i+...G_k^i)^2 d\tau\right]\left[\sum_{j=1}^{M}\sum_{j=1}^{M} q_j q_j \int (G_1^j+G_2^j+...G_k^j)^2 d\tau\right]}}$$

where:

$$G_k^i = \gamma_k e^{-\alpha_k(r-R_i)^2}$$

The integral terms expand into a series of two-center Gaussian overlap integrals. These two-center integrals have a simple form based on exponent values and distances between atom centers [4], for example:

$$\int e^{-\alpha_1(r-R_i)^2} e^{-\alpha_2(r-R_j)^2} d\tau = \left(\frac{\pi}{\alpha_1+\alpha_2}\right)^{3/2} \exp\left(-\frac{\alpha_1\alpha_2}{\alpha_1+\alpha_2}|R_i - R_j|^2\right)$$

It is therefore possible to break down the similarity computation in to a series of readily calculable exponent terms.

These terms can be evaluated extremely quickly, and since no singularity exists as r approaches zero, electrostatic potential evaluations need not be restricted to regions outside the van der Waals radii.

For the index which relates to the repulsive contribution to binding the obvious property is shape. Again the early work [5] in this area computed the shape property numerically using a point counting formulae: a point inside a molecular van der Waals surface was given the value unity while points outside have the value zero. Hence the similarity of shape in the Carbo formalism is simply:

$$\text{Similarity} = \frac{B}{\sqrt{T_A T_B}}$$

With B being the number of points falling inside both molecules and T_A and T_B being the total number of points inside molecule A and B respectively. Once again we can avoid the problems inherent in using coarse grids of points and numerical integration by using a Gaussian approximation of orbital electron density.

Instead of using van der Waals radius data, atomic electron density functions are used to describe the shape of each atom. These functions are determined from the square of the STO3G atomic orbital wave functions [6]. Three Gaussian functions were then fitted to the resulting electron density of each atom type [7]. Rather than using a grid to determine shape similarity, these Gaussian functions are used analytically within the Carbo formula as above. It is then possible to evaluate shape similarity through a series of readily calculable terms [8].

3. Similarity matrices and QSAR. Quantitative structure activity relations play an important part in the application of computational methods to drug design, the aim being to derive a correlation between structural features of molecules and their biological activity. Among the more important approaches to relating molecular properties to observed biological data has been the work of Hopfinger [9,10], who compared differences in fields and molecular volumes, and the widely used method of Cramer et al, based on comparative molecular field analysis (CoMFA) which employs partial least squares statistics [11,12], to analyse the steric and electrostatic fields at lattice points surrounding molecules.

Since much of this type of information is contained within similarity indices they too can form the basis of a simple approach to structure activity relations, both qualitative and quantitative. Typically the medicinal chemist will have produced a series of compounds A, B, C.. etc. We may calculate a matrix of similarity between all pairs of molecules. If there are N molecules in the series this will result in an $N \times N$ matrix of similarity in shape and a similar matrix of electrostatic potential similarity. These may be combined to yield an $N \times 2N$ matrix if so desired.

A qualitative relationship can be extracted from the information using neural network pattern recognition techniques [13,14], or a quantitative relationship using partial least squares. The results are comparable with those obtained with more detailed methods but are much more rapid. That speed however is gained at the expense of a loss of detailed information about sub-molecular contributions.

4. Faster methods, working in two dimensions. A completely new set of demands on similarity calculations has arisen from the advent of combinatorial chemistry and high throughput synthesis. Instead of dealing with tens of compounds the pharmaceutical industry is faced with tens of thousands or even millions of compounds. There is a need to measure how diverse such a set of molecules are and to seek out similarities and structure activity relations. That demands very rapid methods of computation.

One way in which this may be attempted is to reduce the dimensionality of the problem by working in two dimensions. We have shown [15] in the case of proteins that non-linear mapping may be used to produce two- dimensional representations which retain the three dimensional distance information in terms of atom-atom distances to an accuracy of about $3\AA$. We now apply this to give two dimensional representations of small molecules.

Consider a molecule containing N atoms, each of these atoms has a position in three dimensional space which can be represented by a three dimensional position vector $\boldsymbol{P3_i}$. These three dimensional atomic positions can either be acquired from X-ray crystallographic sources, or, to a high degree of accuracy, from a molecular modeling package. We can calculate the distance between the ith and jth element of this list of atom positions using the following equation:

$$D3_{i,j} = \langle\langle \boldsymbol{P3}_i| - \langle \boldsymbol{P3}_j|||\boldsymbol{P3}_i\rangle - |\boldsymbol{P3}_j\rangle\rangle$$

This can be seen to be the square of the Euclidean distance between the atoms. These distances can be compiled into a matrix of three dimensional distances $\boldsymbol{D3}$:

$$\boldsymbol{D3} = \begin{bmatrix} D3_{0,0} & D3_{1,0} & \cdots \\ D3_{0,1} & \cdots & \cdots \\ \cdots & \cdots & D3_{N,N} \end{bmatrix}$$

Now consider forming a N element list of two dimensional position vectors $\boldsymbol{P2}$. These also can be used to form a matrix of two dimensional distances $\boldsymbol{D2}$ whose elements are given by:

$$D2_{i,j} = \langle\langle \boldsymbol{P2}_i| - \langle \boldsymbol{P2}_j|||\boldsymbol{P2}_i\rangle - |\boldsymbol{P2}_j\rangle\rangle$$

In order to preserve the structure of the three dimensional data in the two dimensional data we need to modify the $\boldsymbol{P2}_i$ in such a manner that the elements of the error matrix E are minimized.

$$E_{i,j} = W_{i,j}(D3_{i,j} - D2_{i,j})^2$$

$W_{i,j}$ are the elements of a weighting matrix which describes which distances are the more important. This weighting matrix did not appear in our original work, and is included for flexibility. The method currently implemented is the method of steepest descents, for this we require an expression for the first and second derivatives of the error with respect to each component of the N vectors in $\boldsymbol{P2}$. Such expressions are readily derived and are presented below:

$$\frac{\partial e}{\partial\omega(|\boldsymbol{P2}_i\rangle)} = -4\sum_{j=0}^{N} W_{i,j}(\omega(|\boldsymbol{P2}_i\rangle) - \omega(|\ \boldsymbol{P2}_j\rangle))(D3_{i,j} - D2_{i,j})$$

$$\frac{\partial^2 E}{\partial\omega(|\boldsymbol{P2}\rangle)^2} = \sum_{j=0}^{N} 8W_{i,j}(\omega(|\boldsymbol{P2}_i\rangle) - \omega(|\boldsymbol{P2}_j\rangle))^2 - 4W_{i,j}(D3_{i,j} - D2_{i,j})$$

The function ω extracts the required component from the vector $\boldsymbol{P2}_i$. Then if $\omega(\boldsymbol{P2}_i)$ is the current best value for the component a better estimate, i.e. one which will reduce the error still further, is given by $\omega(\boldsymbol{P2}_i)$ where:

$$\omega(|\boldsymbol{P2}_i\rangle) = \omega(|\boldsymbol{P2}_i\rangle) - \eta\Delta$$
$$\Delta = \ frac\frac{\partial E}{\partial\omega(|\boldsymbol{P2}_i\rangle)}\left|\frac{\partial^2 E}{\partial\omega(|\boldsymbol{P2}_i\rangle)^2}\right|$$

η is an constant which enables some control over the steepest descent minimization process, in the current implementation a value of 0.4 was used with good results.

There is a problem when molecules are quasi-spherical, but for most typical sets of molecules encountered in drug design this is not serious.

The two-dimensional representations provide the basis for very rapid similarity calculations using pattern recognition techniques.

5. Relative configuration space. Even when working in two dimensions it might seem that we still have to expend a lot of time optimizing the superposition which would involve a complete search of relative configuration space. This can however be avoided using a variety of techniques introduced in pattern recognition algorithms.

The technique of invariant moments was introduce by Hu [16]. The method is based upon a statistical analysis of the distribution and value of the pixels which make up the image to be compared. This distribution takes the form of the following equation:

$$m_{p,q} = \int\int x^p y^q \rho(x,y)dxdy \qquad \text{for continuous data.}$$

or

$$m_{p,q} = \sum\sum x^p y^q \rho(x,y) \qquad \text{for discrete data.}$$

Now from a uniqueness theorem due to Papoulis [17] provided that $\rho(x,y)$ is continuous, and has non zero values only in a finite part of the x, y plane, moments of all orders exist and the sequence of moments $m_{p,q}$ are uniquely determined by $\rho(x,y)$. Conversely it can be shown that the infinite sequence of $m_{p,q}$ uniquely determines $\rho(x,y)$.

It should be immediately apparent that the above equations suffer from the same problem as the traditional Carbo index, in that they are sensitive to translation and rotation. These effects can be removed as follows:

Inherent in the equations for generating the moments is the assumption that the property $\rho(x,y)$ is centred upon the calculation co-ordinates. This may not be the case. However let us define two parameters as follows:

$$\overline{x} = \frac{m_{1,0}}{m_{0,0}}$$
$$\overline{y} = \frac{m_{0,1}}{m_{0,0}}$$

These two parameters clearly give the center of the property $\rho(x, y)$ in the calculation co-ordinate system. This has been shown to be consistently positioned for all systems which can be reasonably compared. Then let us define the central moment $\mu_{p,q}$ by the following equation:

$$\mu_{p,q} = \int\int (x - \overline{x})^p (y - \overline{y})^q \rho(x, y) dx dy \text{ for continuous data.}$$

or

$$\mu_{p,q} = \sum\sum (x - \overline{x})^p (y - \overline{y})^q \rho(x, y) \text{ for discrete data.}$$

These central moments have the desired invariance to translation.

For rotational invariance there is a much more complex operation than the above process.

Aligning a structure along its principal axes enables us to remove any unwanted rotation. In the case of the moments Hu utilises this property of the principal axes to rotate $\rho(x, y)$ so that the propertys distribution is aligned along the calculation axes. He does this by forming a variety of combinations of the three second order central moments and the four third order central moments. In his paper Hu explains the logic behind these combinations, which are able to distinguish between structures which exhibit mirror and rotational symmetry:

$$\eta_0 = \mu_{20} + \mu_{02}$$

$$\eta_1 = \sqrt{|(\mu_{20} - \mu_{02})^2 4\mu_{11}^2|}$$

$$\eta_2 = \sqrt{|(\mu_{30} - 3\mu_{12})^2 + (3\mu_{21} - \mu_{03})^2|}$$

$$\eta_3 = \sqrt{|(\mu_{30} - \mu_{12})^2 + (\mu_{21} + \mu_{03})^2|}$$

$$\eta_4 = \sqrt[4]{\left| \begin{array}{l} (\mu_{30} - 3\mu_{12})(\mu_{30} + \mu_{12})[(\mu_{30} + \mu_{12})^2 - 3(\mu_{21} + \mu_{03})^2] + \\ (3\mu_{21} - \mu_{03})(\mu_{21} + \mu_{03})[3(\mu_{30} + \mu_{12})^2 - (\mu_{21} + \mu_{03})^2] \end{array} \right|}$$

$$\eta_5 = !\sqrt[3]{(\mu_{20} - \mu_{02})[(\mu_{30} + \mu_{12})^2 - (\mu_{21} + \mu_{03})^2] + 4\mu_{11}(\mu_{30} + \mu_{12})(\mu_{21} + \mu_{03})}$$

$$\eta_6 = \sqrt[4]{\left| \begin{array}{l} (3\mu_{21} - \mu_{03})(\mu_{30} + \mu_{12})[(\mu_{30} + \mu_{12})^2 - 3(\mu_{21} + \mu_{03})^2] + \\ (3\mu_{12} - \mu_{30})(\mu_{21} + \mu_{03})[3(\mu_{30} + \mu_{12})^2 - (\mu_{21} + \mu_{03})^2] \end{array} \right|}$$

These seven invariant central moments are all that is required to gain a reasonable degree of sensitivity in pattern recognition.

Utilising the invariant central moments is fairly straightforward. All we have to do is to project our molecular property onto a grid and run through the calculations detailed above. This gives us a seven dimensional

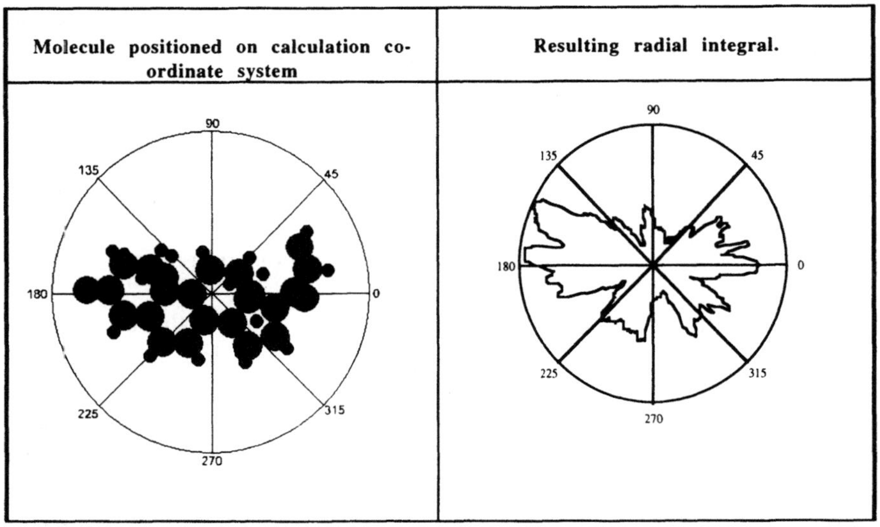

FIG. 1. *Example of a radial integral as applied to a steroid molecule.*

vector $\eta_{A,2D}$ which represents the distribution of $\rho_{A,2D}(x,y)$. The molecule to be compared can also be subjected to the same treatment, remembering that we no longer have to bother aligning A an B to get the correct answer. This yields a second seven element vector $\eta_{B,2D}$. The similarity, or more properly in this case the distance between the two molecules, is then given by the Euclidean distance of these two vectors in seven dimensional space:

$$D_{A,B} = \frac{|\eta_{A,2D} - \eta_{B,2D}|}{\sqrt{|\eta_{A,2D}||\eta_{B,2D}|}}$$

Clearly the above equation can be calculated in a fraction of the time required for the traditional Carbo or Hodgkin indices.

6. Radial integration for similarity calculations. This powerful technique involves us projecting our molecular property $\rho(x,y)$ upon a calculation co-ordinate system. As we have seen before we need not worry about where we perform this projection as any arbitrary offset is easily accounted for by evaluating $\overline{x}$ and $\overline{y}$.

Now that we have centered the property on the calculation co- ordinate system let us proceed to integrate $\rho(x,y)$ along radii moving from the origin to a distance at which the property is deemed to be zero. We then store this value in an array at the offset corresponding to that angle, as illustrated in figure 1:

The radial integral can be mathematically expressed as:

$$R_A(\theta) = \int_0^R \rho_{A,2D}(r,\theta)dr$$

Now to compare two molecules all we have to do is compare their radial integrals. However this is not as simple as perhaps it initially seems for we still have done nothing about the relative orientations of the two molecules. To get around this problem we utilise correlation theory. Correlation theory is based on an equation known as the correlation integral z_{AB}, which in our case can be stated as:

$$z_{AB}(\Delta\theta) = \int R_A(\theta)R_B(\theta + \Delta\theta)d\theta$$

Let us now investigate what this equation means:

$\Delta\theta$ is being used to rotate the radial integral of molecule B around so that comes into and out of alignment with molecule A. When the molecules are perfectly aligned z_{AB} will have its maximum value, therefore all that we have to do is evaluate the correlation integral for all values of $\Delta\theta$, and search for the maximum value. Assuming that we desire an accuracy of $360/N$ degrees for our search this process would appear to be of the order N^2. However the fundamental reason we are carrying out the non linear map is to gain speed in searching through a large database so it makes some sense to see if we can perform the search much faster. It transpires that the method for carrying out the fast search is very simple provided that we make N an integer power of 2. This is illustrated below:

Consider forming the Fourier transform of the correlation integral, which we shall denote as $\boldsymbol{Z}_{AB}(f)$. This yields:

$$\mathbf{Z_{AB}}(f)=\int z_{AB}(\Delta\theta)e^{-i2\pi f A\theta}d\delta\theta=\int\left[\int R_A(\theta)R_B(\theta+\Delta\theta)d\theta\right]e^{-i2\pi f\Delta 0}d\Delta\theta$$

Now let us assume that the order of integration can be changed in the right hand expression:

$$\mathbf{Z_{AB}}(f) = \int R_A(\theta)\left[\int R_B(\theta + \Delta\theta)e^{-i2\pi f\Delta\theta}d\Delta\theta\right]d\theta$$

Writing $\sigma = \theta + \Delta\theta$ we achieve:

$$\mathbf{Z_{AB}}(f) = \int R_A(\theta)\left[\int R_B(\sigma)e^{-i2\pi f(\sigma-\theta)}d\sigma\right]d\theta$$

$$\mathbf{Z_{AB}}(f) = \int R_A(\theta)e^{i2\pi f\theta}\left[\int R_B(\sigma)e^{-2\pi f\sigma}d\sigma\right]d\theta$$

The term in brackets can be seen to be nothing more than the Fourier transform of the radial integral of molecule B thus:

$$\mathbf{Z_{AB}}(f) = \mathbf{R_B}(f)\int R_A(\theta)e^{i2\pi f\theta}d\theta$$

The remaining integral term is simply the complex conjugate of the Fourier transform of the radial integral of molecule $A, \mathbf{R_A}(f)$. Hence we have established the important result that:

$$\mathbf{Z_{AB}}(f) = \mathbf{R_A}^*(f)\mathbf{R_B}(\mathbf{f})$$

This implies that the complete correlation function can be obtained from the inverse Fourier transform of $\mathbf{Z_{AB}}(f)$.

Cooley and Tukey [18], showed that a fast Fourier transform of N data points could be carried out in a process which was of the order $N \log_2(N)$, provided that N was an integer power of two.

Now our process contains two Fourier transforms to calculate $\mathbf{R_A}$ and $\mathbf{R_B}$, one multiplication loop to form $\mathbf{Z_{AB}}$, an inverse Fourier transform to restore $\mathbf{z_{AB}}$ and a straightforward scan to find the maximum value. Which for $N = 512$ represents a twenty fold improvement in computational requirements over a straight evaluation of the correlation integral for all $\Delta\theta$.

Hence if we denote the similarity calculated from radial integrals as S_{AB}^{RI} we can write the following equation:

$$S_{AB}^{RI} = \frac{\max(z_{AB}(\Delta\theta))}{\sqrt{\int R_A^2(\theta)d\theta \int R_B^2(\theta)d\theta}}$$

The denominator, once more, just scales the result to lie between 0 and 1. It adds only complexity $2N$ to the process and is therefore insignificant.

7. Conclusions. The possible applications of pattern recognition methods to similarity are by no means exhausted in this short introductory account and we ourselves have experimented with several other techniques [19]. What is clear however is the need for rapid similarity comparisons and this type of approach has great promise. Ideally we would like to process chemical structures which contain distance information as rapidly as text can now be read by machine.

REFERENCES

[1] R. Carbo, L. Leyda and M. Arnau. An electron density measure of the similarity between two compounds. Int. J. Quantum Chem. 17, 1185–1189 (1980).

[2] E.E. Hodgkin and W.G. Richards. Molecular similarity based on electrostatic potential and electric field. Int. J. Quantum Chem. Quantum Biol. Symp. 14, 105–110 (1987).

[3] A.C. Good, E.E. Hodgkin and W.G. Richards. The utilization of Gaussian functions for the rapid evaluation of molecular similarity. J. Chem. Inf. Comput. Sci. 33, 188–191 (1992).

[4] A. Szabo and N.S. Ostlund. Modern Quantum Chemistry. Macmillan, Basingstoke. 1982. 410–412.

[5] A.M. Meyer and W.G. Richards. Similarity of molecular shape. J. Comput. Aided. Mole. Des. 5, 426–439 (1991).

[6] J. A. Pople et al. Gaussian94. Gaussian Inc. Pitsburgh, PA.

[7] P.E. Gill and W. Murray. Algorithms for the solution of non-linear least squares problems. J. Numer. Anal. 15, 977–982 (1978).

[8] A.C. Good and W.G. Richards. Rapid evaluation of shape similarity using Gaussian functions. J. Chem. Inf. Comput. Sci. 33, 112–116 (1993).

[9] A.J. Hopfinger. A QSAR investigation of DHFR inhibition by Bakers triazines based upon molecular shape analysis. J. Am. Chem. Soc. 102, 7196–7206. (1980).

[10] A.J. Hopfinger. Theory and analysis of molecular potential energy fields in molecular shape analysis: a QSAR study of 2,4-diamino 5-benzylpyrimidines as DHFR inhibitors. J. Med. Chem. 26, 990–996. (1983).

[11] R.D. Cramer, D. E. Patterson and J. D. Bunce. Comparative molecular field analysis (CoMFA) Effect of shape on binding of steroids to carrier proteins. J. Am. Chem. Soc. 110, 5959–5967 (1988).

[12] J. W. McFarland. Comparative molecular field analysis of anticoccidial triazines. J. Med. Chem. 35, 2543–2550. (1992).

[13] A.C. Good, Sung-Sau So and W.G. Richards. Structure activity relationships from molecular similarity matrices. J. Med. Chem. 36, 433–438 (1993).

[14] A.C. Good, S. J. Peterson and W. G. Richards. QSARs from similarity matrices. Technique validation and application in the comparison of different similarity evaluation methods. J. Med. Chem. 36, 2929–2937 (1993).

[15] T.W. Barlow and W. G. Richards. A novel representation of protein structure. J. Molec. Graph. 13, 373-376 (1996).

[16] M. K. Hu. Visual pattern recognition by moment invariants. IRE Transactions on Information Theory. 1962 179–187.

[17] A. Papoulis. Probability, Random variables and Stochastic processes. McGraw-Hill. New York, 1965.

[18] J. W. Cooley and J. W. Tukey. An algorithm for machine calculation of complex Fourier series. Math. Computation. 19, 97–301 (1956).

[19] D. D. Robinson, T. W. Barlow and W. G. Richards. The utilization of reduced dimensional representations of molecular structure for rapid molecular similarity calculations. J. Chem. Inf. Comput. Sci. in press.

MODELING THE EFFECT OF SOLVATION ON STRUCTURE, REACTIVITY, AND PARTITIONING OF ORGANIC SOLUTES: UTILITY IN DRUG DESIGN

CANDEE C. CHAMBERS*, DAVID J. GIESEN†, GREGORY D. HAWKINS‡, CHRISTOPHER J. CRAMER‡, DONALD G. TRUHLAR‡, AND WOUTER H.J. VAES§

Abstract. The SM*x* family of quantum mechanical solvation models accounts for electric and electronic polarization via the generalized Born model and for non-electrostatic components of solvation by microscopic surface tensions. The SM5.4 model, which is the most physical member of the SM*x* family, has been parameterized using two electronic Hamiltonians, AM1 and PM3. For both Hamiltonians, solvation parameters are obtained for water and for any organic solvent for which certain macroscopic data are available, in particular, the index of refraction, bulk surface tension, dielectric constant, and hydrogen bonding acidity and basicity as measured by the Abraham empirical α_2^H and β_2^H scales. For neutral solutes, the mean unsigned errors for aqueous and non-aqueous free energies of solvation are both 0.5 kcal/mol based on 215 and 1786 data points, respectively (for either Hamiltonian). By adding solvation effects to the gas-phase Hamiltonian, it is possible to model the effects of solvent on conformational analysis, molecular recognition, reaction kinetics, etc. The SM5.4 model is also useful for the calculation of solute partitioning between two solvents. Moreover, it is possible to generalize the SM5.4 model to media that are less well characterized than homogeneous solvents—an example is presented here for the case of bilayers of phosphatidyl choline—in order to model partitioning between biophases.

1. Introduction. By their very nature as molecular bullets aimed at (usually macromolecular) targets in condensed-phase systems, drugs, or more accurately their structure and reactivity, can only be realistically modeled within the context of their surroundings. For instance, it is well appreciated within the pharmaceutical industry that *in vitro* activity will not correlate with *in vivo* efficacy if drug delivery is stymied by insolubility in water. Efficiency of transport from one biophase to another, e.g., blood to cell membrane, can also play a critical role in drug bioactivity, and this efficiency is fundamentally related to the ability of the two different phases to differentially solvate the drug [1, 2]. Another example of the role of a drug's surroundings is that interaction of a drug with its target necessitates the desolvation of each over some fraction of their molecular surface areas. If those surfaces interact favorably with the surrounding biophase, the loss of this interaction must reduce binding efficiency.

In principle, all of these effects can be modeled from knowledge of the

*Departments of Physics and Chemistry, Mercyhurst College, 501 E. 38th St., Erie, PA 16546.

†Eastman Kodak Co., 1999 Lake Avenue, Rochester, NY 14650.

‡Department of Chemistry and Supercomputer Institute, 207 Pleasant St. SE, Minneapolis, MN 55455-0431.

§Research Institute of Toxicology, Utrecht University, P.O. Box 80176, NL-3508 TD Utrecht, The Netherlands.

free energies of solvation of the system at relevant sites (e.g., the drug in different phases or the isolated drug and receptor vs. the complex of the two). This chapter will focus on the use of the semiempirical SM5 family of quantum mechanical solvation models to calculate solvation and partitioning free energies for organic solutes. A special advantage of quantum mechanical solvation models is that they can predict the dependence of solvation free energy on conformation. Such information is important for modeling partitioning and binding phenomena, but only rarely is it available from experiment.

Section 2 reviews the functional forms of the models and documents their performance, Section 3 illustrates application of the models to two conformational analysis problems in solution, Section 4 describes the application of the models to compute partition coefficients between water and chloroform and water and a phospholipid bilayer, and Section 5 offers final remarks.

2. The SM5 models. Full descriptions of the SM5 models are presented elsewhere [3–8]. This section reviews those features that are most critical as background for the issues addressed in this chapter. The SM5 models are quantum statistical continuum solvation models. The solvent is modeled as a homogeneous surrounding medium that affects the quantum mechanical self-consistent-field equations for the solute orbitals, and the model includes additional terms designed to account for specific interactions between the solute and its surrounding first solvent shell. For all SM5 models (and for all previous SMx models), the standard-state free energy of solvation is partitioned into two contributions [9–13]

$$\Delta G_S^0 = \Delta G_{ENP} + G_{CDS} \tag{1}$$

where ΔG_{ENP} is the electrostatic component of the solvation free energy, i.e., the change in the electronic and nuclear internal energy of the solute and the electric polarization free energy of the solute-solvent system upon insertion of the solute in the solvent, and G_{CDS} is the contribution of non-electrostatic short- and medium-range effects to the standard-state free energy of transfer. The S in ΔG_S^0 stands for solvation, *ENP* stands for electronic-nuclear-polarization, and *CDS* stands for cavitation-dispersion-solvent-structure. All SM5 models use a standard state of 298 K and 1 M in both the gas phase and solution.

The remainder of Section 2 describes the steps employed to parameterize an SM5 model. That process involves both the *ENP* and the *CDS* terms, and we will discuss the procedure in that order. It is worth emphasizing here, however, that the characteristics that distinguish SM5 models from previous SMx solvation models [9, 14–21] are the use of fixed atomic radii for defining molecular cavities and surfaces of all atoms except (sometimes) hydrogens, the avoidance of strictly empirical modifications of the electrostatics (thereby placing explicitly empirical terms in the *CDS* term rather than the *ENP* term of the equation above), and the use of geometry-dependent atomic surface tensions, as described more fully below.

2.1. Electrostatic components of solvation. The ΔG_{ENP} term can be further partitioned as

$$\Delta G_{ENP} = \Delta E_{EN} + G_P \tag{2}$$

where ΔE_{EN} is the change in the electronic and nuclear energy of the solute in going from the gas phase to solution, and G_P is the electric polarization free energy of the solvent, due to solute-solvent interactions and the change in solvent-solvent interactions upon inserting the solute. In the SM5 models parameterized so far, the terms in equation 2 are calculated using neglect-of-diatomic-differential-overlap molecular orbital theory with either the Austin Model 1 [22–24] (AM1) or Parameterized Model 3 [25] (PM3) Hamiltonian; these choices are distinguished by the notations SM5.../AM1 and SM5.../PM3, respectively, where the ellipses represent additional notation required to fully specify the model (vide infra).

G_P is calculated from the partial atomic charges q_k according to the Generalized Born equation [9, 10, 17, 26–36]

$$G_P = -\frac{1}{2}\left(1 - \frac{1}{\varepsilon}\right) \sum_{k,k'} q_k q_{k'} \gamma_{kk'} \tag{3}$$

where ε is the solvent dielectric constant, k and k' label atoms, and $\gamma_{kk'}$ is a Coulomb integral that accounts for either the self-energy of a charge in a dielectric medium ($k = k'$) or the dielectric screening of the Coulomb interaction of two charges ($k \neq k'$) Additional details of the computation of $\gamma_{kk'}$ are provided in Section 2.1.2, but we note here that a very critical aspect of the screening algorithm is that it allows other parts of the solute to descreen each partial charge in terms of the solvent volume that they displace. Since the partial atomic charges used in equation 3 are derived from the wave function, the Fock operator must be modified to make the total energy, which includes this term, variational [3, 9–13, 20, 30–33, 37]. This is accomplished by including a self-consistent reaction field (SCRF) in the Fock operator of the Hartree-Fock equations. The Fock operator is modified by the dependence of the partial atomic charges on density matrix elements, and the next section discusses this dependence for the different SM5 models.

2.1.1. Partial atomic charges. We have previously identified four classes of partial atomic charges that find use in diverse modeling efforts [16, 38]. These classes are defined as: (I) charges postulated without reference to quantum mechanics, e.g., one might calculate partial charges for a diatomic molecule by dividing its dipole moment by its bond length, (II) charges extracted from a quantum mechanical wave function by analyzing the wave function using *ad hoc* prescriptions—of these, Mulliken population analysis [39] is perhaps the most widely used, (III) charges extracted from a quantum mechanical wave function by analyzing a physical observable *predicted from the wave function*, e.g., the electrostatic potential [40–43] and (IV) methods that map Class II or Class III charges in a manner designed to improve agreement with a physical observable, e.g., the dipole moment [38], *as measured by experiment or converged quantum mechanics*. Different SM5 models are designed to use different classes of partial atomic charges, as further described in the next three sections.

2.1.1.1. SM5.4. The addition of ".4" to "SM5" indicates that the charge model employed for the electrostatic component of the free energy of solvation is a Class IV charge model. All SM5.4 calculations described in this paper are carried out by the SM5.4/AM1 model, in which the CM1A charge model [38], which maps AM1 zero-differential-overlap Mulliken charges to Class IV charges, is employed. (The SM5.4/PM3 solvation model uses the PM3-based charge model, CM1P [38], but is not discussed further here). The CM1 charge models were designed to deliver charges that reproduce gas-phase dipole moments for small neutral solutes as closely as possible [38]. Note that for polar neutral molecules the electrostatic potential at large distances is determined entirely by the dipole moment, so this is a special case of electrostatic potential fitting. Since the charge distribution of a large molecule is determined even at shorter distances primarily by bond dipoles and individual functional groups, a model that works well for dipole moments of small molecules should also work well for charge distributions of large molecules, if the model is properly formulated. The SM5.4 models have been parameterized for water [3, 5] and for any organic solvent for which five readily available descriptors are known, as described in more detail in Section 2.2 below.

In additional work not yet available at the time that this this chapter is being prepared, our group is creating a series of 5.42R models based on AM1, PM3, *ab initio* Hartree-Fock, and density functional theory. These models involve a new class IV charge model called CM2, and are designed to be used with "rigid" gas-phase geometries. To denote these changes we add 2R to the names. We are also considering the preparation of a 5.42 non-rigid model based on AM1 and PM3 with CM2 changes. The SM5.42 models will be preferred to SM5.4 models for several reasons: (1) CM2 charges are more accurate than CM1 charges. (2) The SM5.42 models, coming later than the SM5.4 models, incorporate improvements in the training set, in some of the surface tension functionals, and in the empirical effective solvent radius.

2.1.1.2. SM5.2. The addition of ".2" to "SM5" indicates that the charge model employed for the electrostatic component of the free energy of solvation is a Class II charge model. For all SM5.2 calculations described in this paper, the charges employed are derived from Mulliken population analysis [39] of the zero-differential-overlap AM1 wave function. Although Class II charges are less realistic than Class IV charges, they are more efficient to calculate and do not require new parameterization, so they may serve for instances where system complexity motivates the use of a faster method or for solutes involving atom types for which a Class IV charge model has not yet been parameterized. Models using Class II charges are, however, much less robust for applications to transition states or functional groups that were not included in the training set. The only currently available SM5.2 model is for water [5], and that model (called SM5.2PD/AM1) is only defined for the case where the dielectric descreening is calculated via the pairwise descreening approximation, as described more fully in Section 2.1.2.

A quartet of SM5.2R models with volume descreening are, however, currently being parameterized [8] for both water and organic solvents using the AM1, PM3, MNDO [44], and MNDO/d [45–47] electronic Hamiltonians and will probably be available by the time these proceedings are published. These models are called SM5.2R/AM1, SM5.2R/PM3, SM5.2R/MNDO, and SM5.2R/MNDO/d, where "R" again denotes that the solute geometry is rigid, i.e., not re-optimized in solution. The rigid models are parameterized using gas-phase geometrics. Thus geometry relaxation in solution is modeled only in an average implicit way through the parameters.

2.1.1.3. SM5.0R. The addition of ".0" to "SM5" indicates that *no* charge model is employed for the electrostatic component of the free energy of solvation, i.e., all charges are set to zero and consequently G_P is also zero (in fact, ΔG_{ENP} is zero) [8]. Thus, in the parameterization of an SM5.0R model, the model depends on the Hamiltonian only to the extent that different Hamiltonians predict different molecular geometries—there is no dependence on electronic density matrix elements through partial atomic charges. Furthermore, the total free energy of solvation is carried in the CDS term as described in Section 2.2 below, and this term is calculated without reoptimizing the gas-phase geometry in solution, although the empirical nature of the parameters make up for this computational restraint; we call the model SM5.0R to denote this "rigid" aspect. While the SM5.0R assumptions are not particularly physical, since they correspond to modeling long-range electrostatic effects entirely in terms of short-range functions involving surface areas, and since the geometry *does* change upon dissolution, the method can deliver high predictive accuracy for solutes with functional groups similar to those in the parameterization set, and calculation of the solvation free energy is extremely rapid given a previously obtained molecular geometry. All SM5.0R calculations described in this paper are for AM1 solute geometries and all solutes are uncharged. A modification of the SM5.0R model, SM5.05R, exists to handle certain kinds of charged solutes typically found in proteins, and interested readers are referred to the original paper for details [8].

2.1.2. Dielectric descreening. The polarization energy of a system comprised of two charged spheres in a homogeneous dielectric continuum can be solved analytically, but that ceases to be the case upon the introduction of one or more additional spheres. If the solute is represented as a union of partially charged atomic spheres, accounting for the dielectric descreening that results from having additional solute atoms displace the dielectric medium must either be accomplished by solving the Poisson equation or by an approximation to this procedure [13]. The Generalized Born approach employs the latter method, calculating $\gamma_{kk'}$ in equation 3 by an empirical algorithm that accounts for descreening of solute atoms, i.e., displacement of a volume of the dielectric continuum by the remaining molecular volume of the solute [9, 17, 35] generalized Born model replaces the solvation of a differential equation (Poisson's equation) by a quadrature. It involves determining effective atomic radii by a numerical integration of the free energy density surrounding each solute atom assuming that all other solute atoms displace the dielectric medium and assuming that the free energy density is given by Coulomb's law for a single charge in the medium. It employs these radii in an empirical form for $\gamma_{kk'}$. Unless otherwise specified, it is this approach that is used for any SM5 model having non-zero ΔG_{ENP}.

An alternative method to calculate the dielectric descreening is to take advantage of the analytic form available for a system of two spheres, and to assume that the descreening of any solute atom can be calculated by summing all pairwise descreenings owing to other solute atoms [5, 18, 48]. Such an approach ignores overlap between the descreening spheres (i.e., some descreening will be counted multiple times because the descreened volume is shared by multiple spheres), but by scaling the atomic radii to compensate it is possible to account for that overlap in an average way. Such a descreening approach is referred to here as "pairwise descreening", and is abbreviated PD. The SM5.2 models discussed below all employ the pairwise descreening approximation and the AM1 Hamiltonian, and are properly referred to as SM5.2PD/AM1 [5]. SM5.4PD models are also available [5].

2.2. Non-electrostatic components of solvation. As noted above, the non-electrostatic components of the solvation free energy are largely associated with interactions of the solute with its first solvation shell. In SMx models they are assumed to be proportional to the area of a surface through that shell. Thus, the SM5 first-solvation-shell term has the general form:

$$G_{CDS} = \sum_k \sigma_k A_k(R_S^{CD}) + \sigma^{CS} \sum_k A_k(R_S^{CS}) \tag{4}$$

where k denotes an atom, $A_k(R_S^{CX})$ is the solvent-accessible surface area [17, 49] of atom k as calculated for a solvent effective radius R_S^{CX}, σ_k is the atomic surface tension (a surface tension is any quantity having units of energy per unit area), and σ^{CS} is a molecular surface tension calculated for a solvent effective radius R_S^{CS}. In the SM5.4 and SM5.2 models parameterized so far, $R_S^{CD} = R_S^{CS} = 1.7$ Å in water, and $R_S^{CD} =$

$R_S^{CS}/2 = 1.7$ Å in organic solvents. In the SM5.0R and SM5.05R models, we take $R_S^{CD} = R_S^{CS} = 0$. This reduces the solvent-accessible surface area to the van der Waals surface area. The atomic surface tensions depend upon the local geometry of the solute and one or more composite surface tension coefficients $\hat{\sigma}_Z, \hat{\sigma}_{ZZ'}$ and $\hat{\sigma}_{ZZ'}^{(2)}$ that are themselves dependent on the atomic numbers Z and Z' of the atoms and are parameters of the model. The set of functions describing these dependencies are part of what defines a model as being of the SM5 variety, and they have been described in detail [3–6]. The molecular surface tension σ^{CS} is a constant for a given solvent.

We note that in the parameterization of all SM5 models except the R models, solute geometries and electronic wave functions were allowed to fully relax in response to the surrounding solvent. All surface tension coefficients are different (separately optimized) for SM5.4/AM1 and SM5.4/PM3, but all other parameters are the same for the /AM1 and /PM3 cases. We note again that we will discuss only /AM1 models in this chapter.

In the special case of water, since the solvent radii R_S^{CD} and R_S^{CS} are both taken to be 1.7 Å equation 4 simplifies to

$$G_{CDS} = \sum_k \sigma_k A_k(R_S). \tag{5}$$

As a consequence, σ^{CS} is not a separately optimized parameter in the SM5 water models, but is absorbed into the optimization of the atomic surface tension coefficients contributing to each σ_k. The parameterization procedure for water involves calculation of the electrostatic component of the free energy of solvation for a large number of solutes for which experimental data are available, subtracting this value from the experimental free energy of solvation, and optimizing, by linear regression, values for the atomic surface tensions. Details on the performance of the water models can be found in the next section.

In the case of organic solvents, it is uncommon for a single solvent to have sufficient data available to effect a parameterization along the lines of the water models. We addressed this challenge by making the atomic surface tensions themselves be parametric functions of certain macroscopic *solvent* properties; this ensures that the model can be employed for *all* organic solvents for which those properties are available or estimable. To accomplish this, the surface tensions appearing in equation 4 are calculated as

$$\sigma^{CS} = \hat{\sigma}^{CS,n} n + \hat{\sigma}^{CS,\gamma} \gamma \tag{6}$$

$$\tilde{\sigma}_Z = \hat{\sigma}_Z^{(n)} n + \hat{\sigma}_Z^{(\alpha)} \alpha + \hat{\sigma}_Z^{(\beta)} \beta \tag{7}$$

$$\tilde{\sigma}_{ZZ'} = \hat{\sigma}_{ZZ'}^{(n)} n + \hat{\sigma}_{ZZ'}^{(\alpha)} \alpha + \hat{\sigma}_{ZZ'}^{(\beta)} \beta \tag{8}$$

and

$$\bar{\sigma}^{(2)}_{ZZ'} = \hat{\sigma}^{(2,n)}_{ZZ'} n \tag{9}$$

where n is the solvent index of refraction,γ is the macroscopic solvent surface tension, in units of cal mol^{-1} Å^{-2}, and α and β are Abraham's [50–52] indices of solvent hydrogen bonding acidity and basicity, respectively (more specifically, these are the $\sum \alpha_2^H$ and $\sum \beta_2^H$ values for a solvent molecule were it to be taken as a *solute* in the Abraham model). The solvent radii R_S^{CD} and R_S^{CS} are taken to be 1.7 and 3.4 Å, respectively. Two radii were used in order to capture both short-range (cavitation-dispersion) and intermediate-range (cavitation-solvent-structure) effects. Equations 6–9 are used directly for all solvents in the SM5.42R, SM5.2R, and SM5.0R models, and in the SM5.4 models they are used for all solvents except chloroform, benzene, and toluene solvents. In the latter three cases, further adjustments were made to the parameters, and all calculations for these solvents include those adjustments.

2.3. Performance of the SM5 models. Table 1 provides information on the data sets used for parameterization of the various models, and Table 2 provides information on the accuracies of the various models broken down by chemical functionality of solute molecules. Although the SM5.0R, SM5.2PD/AM1, SM5.4PD/AM1, and SM5.4/AM1 models all offer similar accuracy by comparison to experiment, they differ in the degree to which the *ENP* and *CDS* components of the total solvation free energy can be regarded as physical. The level of interpretability is inversely correlated with computational speed, with SM5.4/AM1 being most physical but also most time-consuming, followed by SM5.4PD/AM1, which maintains the use of Class IV charges but approximates the descreening via the pairwise approach, followed by SM5.2PD/AM1 which further approximates the electrostatics by using Class II Mulliken charges, followed at last by SM5.0R, which does not make any attempt to separate electrostatic and non-electrostatic effects, but which is extremely rapid for the computation of solvation free energies, since an electronic structure calculation is not required; rather, for a given geometry, one simply requires a calculation of the solvent exposed surface area.

We now proceed to employ our most physical solvation model, SM5.4/AM1, for the calculation of solvent effects on conformational analysis (next section) and for the computation of partition coefficients (Section 4). In the latter instance, we illustrate how the model may be generalized to media not well described as homogeneous liquid solutions.

3. Solvent effects on conformational analysis. When a solute has multiple low-energy conformations, the population of those conformations at equilibrium is determined by their relative energies in a Boltzmann-

TABLE 1
Data employed in the parameterization of the SM5.4/AM1 model for aqueous and organic solvents and the SM5.4PD/AM1, and SM5.2PD/AM1 models for aqueous solvent.

Solute class	Water number of data	Nonaqueous Solvents number of solutes	number of solvent classes[b]	number of data
unbranched alkanes	8	9	15	76
branched alkanes	5	5	2	7
cycloalkanes	5	4	4	13
alkenes	9	8	3	18
alkynes	5	5	2	9
arenes	8	9	15	126
alcohols	16	17	15	369
ethers	9	9	15	71
aldehydes	6	7	5	32
ketones	12	12	14	191
carboxylic acids	5	5	11	119
esters	12	12	6	227
aliphatic amines	15	11	8	153
aromatic amines	10	11	10	71
nitriles	4	4	4	18
nitrohydrocarbons	6	6	6	32
amides	3[b]	1	3	4
thiols	4	3	3	10
organic sulfides	4	4	3	10
disulfides	2	2	2	3
nonhalobifunctional	8	6	6	26
fluorohydrocarbons	3	5	3	13
chlorohydrocarbons	16	14	4	58
bromohydrocarbons	10	10	4	30
iodohydrocarbons	8	9	4	20
polyfunctional halocarbons	17	13	7	44
inorganic compounds	5	5	9	36
all solutes	215	206	5	1786

[a] For the parameterization of the SM5.0R model for water several additional solute data were added: one urea and several halogenated compounds.

[b] Solvent classes are defined as alkanes, arenes, alcohols, ketones, esters, ethers, amines, pyridines, nitriles, nitrohydrocarbons, tertiary amides, haloaliphatics, haloaromatics, miscellaneous acidic solvents, and miscellaneous non-acidic solvents (15 total solvent classes).

TABLE 2
Mean unsigned error (kcal/mol) for various SM5 models by class of solute[a].

Solute class	Aqueous				Nonaqueous
	SM5.0R	SM5.2PD /AM1	SM5.4PD /AM1	SM5.4 /AM1	SM5.4 /AM1
unbranched alkanes	0.5	0.2	0.5	0.6	0.4
branched alkanes	0.3	0.2	0.3	0.7	0.4
cycloalkanes	0.5	0.2	0.2	0.2	1.0
alkenes	0.2	0.4	0.6	0.5	0.5
alkynes	0.1	0.2	0.2	0.3	0.3
arenes	0.5	0.2	0.2	0.1	0.3
alcohols	0.3	0.4	0.4	0.5	0.4
ethers	0.7	0.5	0.5	0.8	0.4
aldehydes	0.3	0.3	0.3	0.3	0.5
ketones	0.4	0.4	0.2	0.4	0.4
carboxylic acids	0.5	0.7	1.0	0.8	0.6
esters	0.3	0.6	0.7	0.4	0.5
aliphatic amines	0.5	0.5	0.7	0.8	0.4
aromatic amines	1.0	0.6	0.7	0.7	0.4
nitriles	0.6	0.3	0.4	0.5	0.4
nitrohydrocarbons	0.4	0.4	0.5	0.5	0.5
amides	2.8	1.2	1.5	1.8	1.1
thiols	0.3	0.6	0.4	0.3	0.4
organic sulfides	0.3	0.7	0.4	0.4	0.4
disulfides	0.1	0.4	0.3	0.2	0.0
nonhalobifunctional	0.8	0.7	0.5	0.4	0.9
fluorohydrocarbons	1.1	0.4	0.4	0.5	0.4
chlorohydrocarbons	0.5	0.5	0.4	0.4	0.3
bromohydrocarbons	0.4	0.5	0.2	0.2	0.3
iodohydrocarbons	0.9	0.4	0.1	0.2	0.2
polyfunctional halocarbons	0.9	0.7	0.5	0.5	0.6
inorganic compounds	0.8	1.7	1.7	1.8	1.4
all solutes	0.6	0.5	0.5	0.5	0.5

[a] All calculations for AM1 Hamiltonian. These errors do include the additional data mentioned in footnote a of Table 1.

weighted sense. The fraction of the molecules found in conformation A is

$$F(A) = \frac{e^{-G_A^0/RT}}{\sum_i e^{-G_i^0/RT}} \tag{10}$$

where G_A^0 is the free energy of conformer A, and R and T are the universal gas constant and the temperature, respectively.

Since different conformers may have different interactions with the surrounding solvent (because of different charge distributions or different degrees of exposure of solvophobic or solvophilic surface area, for example) the equilibrium distribution of conformers is typically modified by solvation (i.e., the relative G_A^0 values of various conformers may be different in the gas phase than in solution). The SMx solvation models have previously been used to investigate aspects of the aqueous conformational equilibria of heterocycles (where tautomeric equilibria have also been extensively studied) [13, 53–55], sugars [19, 56], cocaine [57], HIV protease inhibitors [58], neurotransmitters [59], nitroaromatic radical anions [60], 1,3-dimethylthiourea [61], 1,2-ethanediol [62], diazene [63], and allyl vinyl ether [64]. The next two sections discuss aspects of the anomeric equilibrium of D-glucose in water and the *gauche/anti* equilibrium of 1,2-dichloroethane in multiple solvents, both being modeled using the SM5.4 method.

3.1. Conformational isomerism of D-glucose. Portions of the conformational potential energy surface for D-glucose have been studied by many researchers [19, 56, 65–76]. The significant conformational issues addressed in these studies revolve around one or more of the following questions: (1) What is the preferred configuration at the anomeric center, and how much higher in energy is the other anomer? (2) What are the preferred orientations of the exocyclic hydroxyl and hydroxymethyl substituents? (3) What is the energetic separation between the two possible chair forms? (4) What are the energetic consequences that arise from the coupling of different conformational issues, e.g., to what extent can one consider the anomeric equilibrium as separate from the hydroxymethyl conformation? (5) How does a surrounding solvent change the intrinsic (gas-phase) conformational preferences? In particular, for hydrogen-bond donor and/or acceptor solvents, to what extent do intermolecular hydrogen bonds between glucose and the solvent compete with intramolecular hydrogen bonds between different glucose hydroxyl groups?

Figure 1 presents the relative free energies for six glucose conformers (three hydroxymethyl rotamers of each anomer) in the gas phase and in aqueous solution. The gas phase results are derived from composite calculations including examination of basis set effects up to valence quadruple zeta, electron correlation effects through coupled cluster with single and double substitutions, geometry optimization using second-order perturbation theory, and thermochemical corrections using the standard rigid-rotor, harmonic oscillator approach [77]. This composite approach is described in greater detail elsewhere [19, 78]. The aqueous relative energies are derived by adding SM5.4/AM1 aqueous solvation free energies to the gas-phase values at the best gas-phase geometries. (Thus we make the approximation of neglecting geometry-relaxation effects in solution.) In both the gas phase and solution, the energy of the αG conformer is taken as 0, and other free energies are relative to this. The bottom rows of the table correspond to the average over the 3 conformations, calculated using equation 10, and to the experimental result; both these rows are relative to the α case, which is arbitrarily set to 0.

As is evident from Figure 1, the experimentally known [79] free energy of anomerization, 0.3 kcal/mol for the $\alpha \rightarrow \beta$ process, is well predicted by the SM5.4/AM1 calculations, which agree with experiment within 0.2 kcal/mol, and the effect of solvation is predicted to stabilize the beta anomer by 0.8 kcal/mol relative to the alpha anomer.

Although this example is averaged over only six conformers, more complete surveys of conformational space using classical mechanical models are entirely consistent with an anomeric solvation effect of this magnitude [73]. The SM5.4/AM1 model has also been used to examine the effect of aqueous solvation on other aspects of glucose conformational analysis [80].

The calculations in Figure 1 are particularly satisfying because they are based on combining state-of-the-art gas-phase calculations with a carefully parameterized solvation model. Previous attempts to understand this issue often suffered from deficiencies in the gas-phase relative free energy as well as from difficulties in the solvation calculation. Another point worth stressing in this example is that SM5.4 models do not suffer from having to make *ad hoc* assumptions about the dependence of partial atomic charges on torsional angles or on the presence of solvent; in SM5.4 models these charges are predicted naturally as an intrinsic part of the self-consistent-field calculation.

3.2. Internal rotational isomerism of 1,2-dichloroethane. As a disubstituted ethane, 1,2-dichloroethane can adopt two equilibrium conformers that differ as rotamers about the *C-C* bond. One rotamer places the two chlorines *trans* to each other (and by symmetry this conformer has a dipole moment of zero), and the other places the two chlorines *gauche* to each other. One would expect the electrostatic interactions of the *gauche* conformer with the dielectric medium to be greater in magnitude than those of the *trans* conformer, because of the finite dipole moment for the former. Of course, other moments play a role as well, and the generalized Born approach accounts for these (unlike, say, the Kirkwood-Onsager model [13, 81, 82], which, by truncating the electronic distribution at the dipole moment, would predict an electrostatic free energy of solvation for the *trans* conformer of zero in all solvents). Non-electrostatic effects will also be different for the two conformers. Table 3 compares the predicted solvent-induced shifts in the *gauche/trans* equilibrium to experiment [83] for eight organic solvents. Agreement is within 0.07 kcal/mol for all solvents except benzene and diethyl ether, where the error is 0.22 and 0.14 kcal/mol, respectively.

This example illustrates the quantitative applicability of the SM5.4/AM1 model to conformational equilibria both in a single solvent and also across multiple solvents. We anticipate that these models will prove useful in examining conformational equilibria for drug molecules, both for understanding their binding and also for modeling their partitioning from one phase to another, as described more fully in the following section.

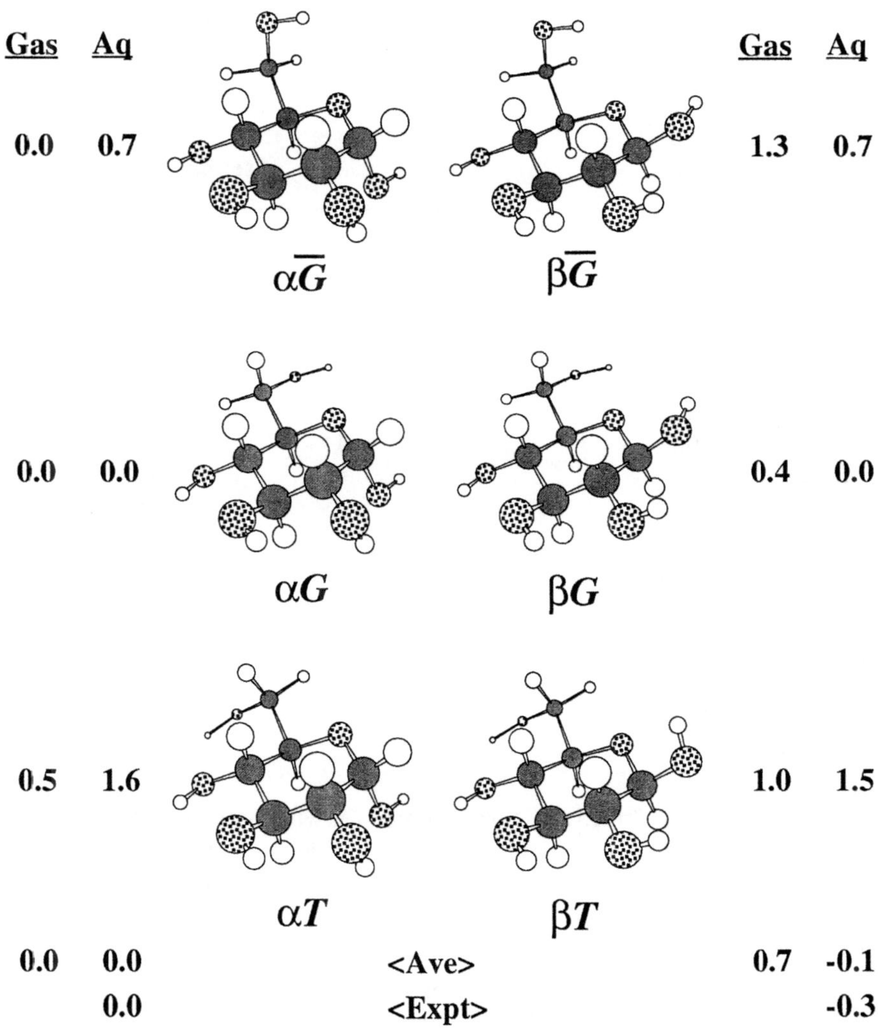

FIG. 1. *Relative free energies (kcal/mol) in the gas phase and in aqueous solution for six glucose conformers (identified as α or β and T, G, or $\bar{G}$ hydroxymethyl rotamers). Gas-phase free energies were calculated from a composite scheme using basis sets up to cc-pVQZ, accounting for electron correlation at the CCSD level, and vibrational frequencies from the HF/cc-pVDZ level. Aqueous free energies were derived by adding SM5.4/AM1 solvation free energies, calculated without geometry relaxation, to the gas-phase values.*

TABLE 3
Magnitude of the solvent-induced shift (kcal/mol) in the gauche/trans equilibrium of 1,2-dichloroethane relative to the gas phase.

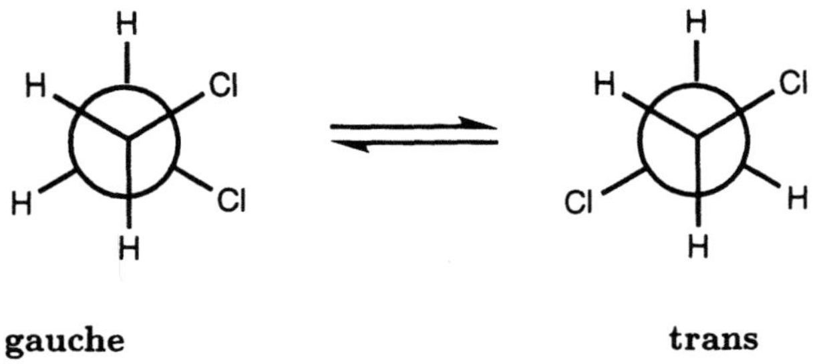

	$\Delta\Delta G_S^0$	
Solvent	SM5.4/AM1	Experimental[a]
Tetrachloroethylene	0.38	0.31
Carbon disulfide	0.44	0.37
Diethyl ether	0.65	0.51
Benzene	0.38	0.60
Ethyl acetate	0.76	0.78
1,2-Dichloroethane (neat liquid)	0.87	0.89
Acetone	0.96	1.02
Acetonitrile	1.00	1.05

[a] Reference [83].

4. Solute partitioning. Solute molecules will partition between multiple phases so as to equalize the concentration-dependent chemical potential of the solute in all phases [84–86]. This behavior affects the bioactivity of the solute. For example, a drug may have very high specific activity against a target enzyme, but if its concentration in aqueous biophases or fatty tissues is extremely low it may not be suitable for oral delivery (since it must be carried by the bloodstream, and it must pass through a lipid bilayer membrane to be absorbed in the small intestine). This illustrates the practical importance of being able to predict concentrations of solutes in different media.

The following two sections focus on the partitioning of solutes between two homogeneous liquid solutions (chloroform and water) and between water and a phospholipid bilayer. Prior studies using the SMx models to correlate solute partitioning between two phases have also appeared [6, 87–90].

TABLE 4
$\log P_{c/w}$ *predicted by two different methods vs. experiment.*

	$\log P_{c/w}$		
	SM5.4/AM1[a]	Reynolds[b]	Experiment[c]
benzene	2.7	4.3	2.8
toluene	3.3	5.0	3.1
ethylbenzene	3.9	5.5	3.7
methanol	−2.0	−1.5	−1.3
ethanol	−0.9	−0.5	−0.9
2-methylpropan-1-ol	0.7	1.0	0.3
1-pentanol	1.1	1.1	1.1
phenol	0.4	1.0	0.4
1-hexanol	1.6	1.6	1.7
1-napthol	2.2[d]	2.3	1.2
ethanal	−0.7	−0.6	0.1
propanone	0.1	1.6	0.4
methyl phenyl ketone	2.3	3.5	2.4
ethanoic acid	−1.3	−1.4	−1.4
butanoic acid	0.2	−0.1	−0.3
hexanoic acid	1.6	1.0	1.0
p-toluic acid	1.8	1.4	1.4
methylamine	−1.5	−0.6	−1.0
diethylamine	1.4	2.8	0.9
pyridine	0.5	2.1	1.3
benzonitrile	3.0	3.1	2.3
2-propen-1-ol	−0.4	0.1	−0.5
ethanamide	−2.2	−3.6	−2.0
chlorobenzene	3.1	4.4	3.2
bromobenzene	3.2	4.3	3.4
p-bromophenol	1.0	0.8	1.1
p-hexylpyridine	4.4	5.4	5.0
propanamide	−1.2	−2.7	−1.4
m-chlorophenol	0.9[d]	0.9	1.0
p-chlorophenol	0.9	0.9	1.0
Mean signed error	0.00	0.44	
Mean unsigned error	0.32	0.73	
Root-mean-square error	0.42	0.95	

[a] Reference [6]. [b] Reference [91]. [c] Reference [92]. [d] Statistically averaged for two hydroxyl rotamers.

4.1. Partitioning between two homogeneous liquids. A reasonable number of data are available for the partitioning of an organic solute between chloroform and water. Reynolds [91] has emphasized the utility of water/chloroform partition coefficients for correlating membrane permeability and bioactivity that depends on this permeability. Reynolds [91] has developed this correlation based on calculations using the GB/SA model of Still *et al.*, [35] which is a nonpolarizable molecular mechanics model with fixed charges and a single molecular surface tension. Table 4 compares the performance of our SM5.4/AM1 models [6] to that of Renolds' calculations [91] for the training set he used to parameterize a subsequent quantitative structure-activity relationship for lipophilicity. The polarizable SM5.4/AM1 models outperform the classical model for the 30 solutes considered by Reynolds. Of these 30 molecules, the first 23 in Table 4 were included in the SM5.4/AM1 Nonaqueous Solvent Parameterization Set (described in Table 1 above), but the remaining 7 molecules were not included in the parameterization set. The results in Table 4 show that the latter molecules are treated with equivalent accuracy. In particular, the mean unsigned error for the first 23 molecules is 0.31 kcal/mol, whereas the mean unsigned error for the last 7 is 0.37 kcal/mol.

4.2. Partitioning between water and phosphatidyl choline bilayers. Although the SM5.4 model for organic solvents was parameterized using data for 90 commonly available solvents, there is every reason to expect that the model will be applicable to *any* condensed phase that has liquid-like properties, e.g., a lipid membrane above its melting temperature. In such an instance, of course, it is not obvious how to go about choosing "correct" values of ε, n, γ, α and β, as are required to define an organic SM5.4 model. However, the solvation free energy as calculated at the SM5.4 level is multilinear in the latter four parameters. A practical approach to dealing with such ill-defined systems is to treat these latter four parameters as fitting parameters—but because the solvation free energy is non-linear in ε, it is more practical to fix this value at some best estimate.

An example of this approach is illustrated for the case of water/phosphatidyl choline unilamellar bilayer partitioning. Experimental partitioning data in this system are available [93] for the solutes illustrated in Figure 2. In the case of phosphatidyl choline, the dielectric constant is unknown; it is probably not unreasonable to assume an effective value that is intermediate between methyl nonadecanoate ($\varepsilon = 3.0$) [94] and tricresyl phosphate ($\varepsilon = 6.7$) [94], and so we used a value of 5. We further assumed that the α value is zero (there are no hydrogen bond donor groups in this molecule), and we regressed the experimental partition coefficients on the remaining three solvent parameters, namely n, γ, and β, employing the AM1 electronic Hamiltonian for the solutes. The regression provides values of 1.40, 27, and 1.15, respectively for these parameters. Such parameter values are very much in keeping with what one might expect based on

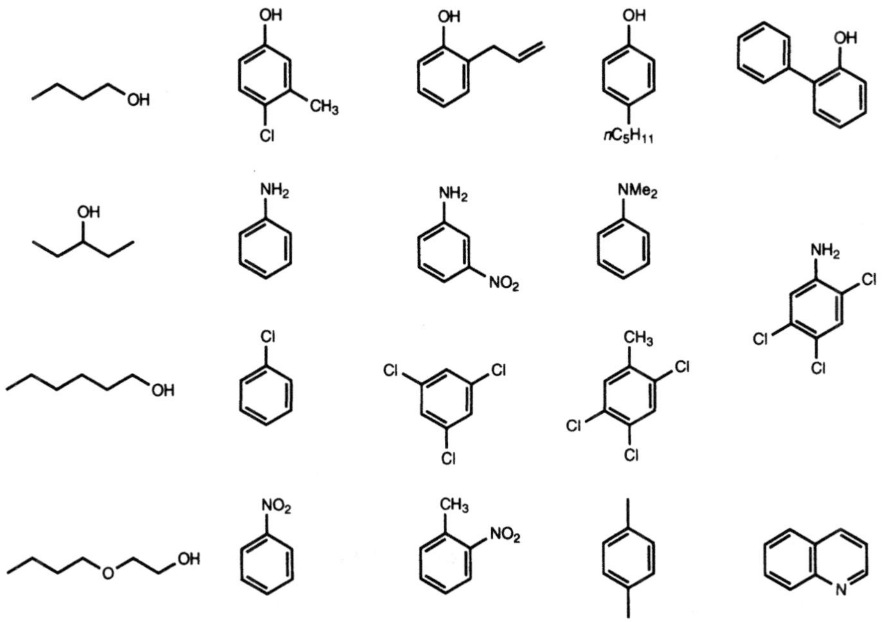

FIG. 2. *Organic solutes for which water/phosphatidyl choline bilayer partitioning data are available.*

analogous molecules as solvents. The regression was also allowed to have a constant term, which is calculated to be 0.59 log units. The quality of the regression, which has an R^2 correlation coefficient of 0.80, is illustrated in Figure 3.

The finding of a constant term in the regression is probably attributable to the amphiphilic nature of several of the solutes. The free energy of solvation calculated by our model for phosphatidyl choline corresponds to complete immersion of the solute in a homogeneous phosphatidyl choline medium. However, many of the experimental solutes presumably maintain hydrophilic contact with the aqueous phase, but bury hydrophobic surface in the lipid phase. This makes the solutes undetectable to the experimental [93] analytic method (which involves microsyringe sampling of an aqueous phase in which the phosphatidyl choline bilayers are suspended), and this makes it appear that the solutes are more soluble in the bilayer than they really are. A more refined model of this process would be one in which a planar boundary separates two homogeneous dielectric media, and this would permit an examination of solute behavior near or at the interface. However, the model presented here is expected to have general utility for the examination of solute partitioning between phases that would otherwise not easily be characterized as solvents, per se.

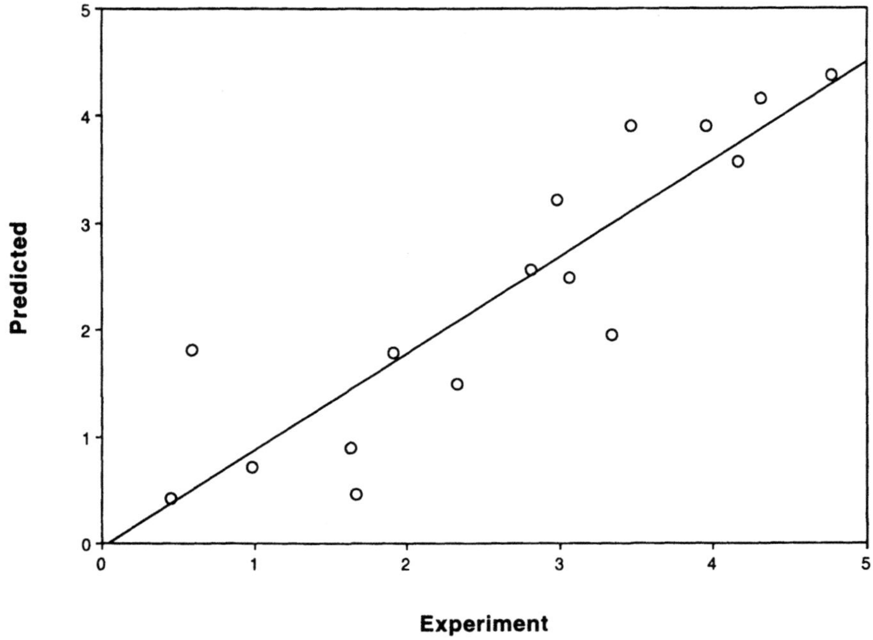

FIG. 3. *Predicted phosphatidyl choline bilayer/water partition coefficients (defined as [molar concentration in phosphatidyl choline bilayer]/ [molar concentration in water] in* $\log_{10}$ *units) vs. experiment for the organic solutes in Figure 2.*

This example illustrates a very general approach to using the SMx models for drug design, an approach that we have labeled as the SRP approach to denote specific reaction parameters or specific range parameters. In this approach we adopt the general framework of the model and most of its parameters from a general parameterization (e.g., in the present case the Coulomb radii, van der Waals radii, and surface tensions were taken from the general SM5.4/AM1 model, but a few parameters (in this case solvent parameters) are adjusted to a specific small data set on a limited range of molecules, e.g., a lead molecule and selected analogs. Having done this, the model could be used for computational screening of other lead analogs as a guide to which ones are most likely to be worthwhile for synthesis. The SRP approach has also been used in other contexts [16, 19, 95–97] and we anticipate it could be extremely powerful for rational drug design.

5. Concluding remarks. SM5 solvation models are designed to offer flexibility to the user in terms of choosing a model based on a balance of speed and interpretability. For neutral organic solutes for which experimental free energies of transfer from the gas phase to a solvent are available, the models typically have mean unsigned errors on the order of 0.5 kcal/mol. When examining solvent effects in individual systems, these errors can cancel out for similar solutes (e.g., conformational isomers) permitting very accurate calculations of solvent effects on conformational equilibria. Furthermore, by being able to calculate free energies of solvation in multiple solvents, it is possible to calculate free energies of partitioning between solvents in a highly accurate fashion. Finally, the SM5.4 model for organic solvents lends itself to specific parameterization for more complicated condensed phases, like lipid bilayers. We anticipate that several of these latter features will make the models useful tools in drug discovery and development.

Acknowledgments. We are grateful for high-performance vector and parallel computing resources made available by the Minnesota Supercomputer Institute and the University of Minnesota-IBM Shared Research Project, respectively. This work was supported by the National Science Foundation, the U.S. Army Research Office, and the Alfred P. Sloan Foundation.

REFERENCES

[1] HANSCH, C.; FUJITA, T., *J. Am. Chem. Soc.*, 1964, **86**, 1616.
[2] SILVERMAN, R.B., *The Organic Chemistry of Drug Design and Drug Action*, Academic: San Diego, 1992, 26–34.
[3] CHAMBERS, C.C.; HAWKINS, G.D.; CRAMER, C.J.; TRUHLAR, D.G., *J. Phys. Chem.*, 1996, **100**, 16385.
[4] GIESEN, D.J.; GU, M.Z.; CRAMER, C.J.; TRUHLAR, D.G., *J. Org. Chem.*, 1996, **61**, 8720.
[5] HAWKINS, G.D.; CRAMER, C.J.; TRUHLAR, D.G., *J. Phys. Chem.*, 1996, **100**, 19824.
[6] GIESEN, D.J.; CHAMBERS, C.C.; CRAMER, C.J.; TRUHLAR, D.G., *J. Phys. Chem.*, 1997, **101**, 2061.
[7] GIESEN, D.J.; HAWKINS, G.D.; LIOTARD, D.A.; CRAMER, C.J.; TRUHLAR, D.G., *Theor. Chem. Acc.*, in press.
[8] HAWKINS, G.D.; CRAMER, C.J.; TRUHLAR, D.G., to be published.
[9] CRAMER, C.J.; TRUHLAR, D.G., *J. Am. Chem. Soc.*, 1991, **113**, 8305.
[10] CRAMER, C.J.; TRUHLAR, D.G., *J. Comput.-Aid. Mol. Des.*, 1992, **6**, 629.
[11] CRAMER, C.J.; TRUHLAR, D.G., In *Quantitative Treatments of Solute/Solvent Interactions*; Politzer, P. and Murray, J.S., Eds.; Elsevier: Amsterdam, 1994, **1**, 9.
[12] CRAMER, C.J.; TRUHLAR, D.G., In *Reviews in Computational Chemistry*; Lipkowitz, K.B. and Boyd, D.B., Eds.; VCH: New York, 1995, **6**, 1.
[13] CRAMER, C.J.; TRUHLAR, D.G., In *Solvent Effects and Chemical Reactivity*; Tapia, O. and Bertrán, J., Eds.; Kluwer: Dordrecht, 1996, 1.
[14] CRAMER, C.J.; TRUHLAR, D.G., *Science*, 1992, **256**, 213.
[15] CRAMER, C.J.; TRUHLAR, D.G., *J. Comp. Chem.*, 1992, **13**, 1089.
[16] STORER, J.W.; GIESEN, D.J.; HAWKINS, G.D.; LYNCH, G.C.; CRAMER, C.J.; TRUHLAR, D.G.; LIOTARD, D.A., In *Structure and Reactivity in Aqueous Solution*; Cramer, C.J. and Truhlar, D.G., Eds.; American Chemical Society: Washington, DC, 1994, 24.
[17] LIOTARD, D.A.; HAWKINS, G.D.; LYNCH, G.C.; CRAMER, C.J.; TRUHLAR, D.G., *J. Comp. Chem.*, 1995, **16**, 422.
[18] HAWKINS, G.D.; CRAMER, C.J.; TRUHLAR, D.G., *Chem. Phys. Lett.*, 1995, **246**, 122.

[19] BARROWS, S.E.; DULLES, F.J.; CRAMER, C.J.; TRUHLAR, D.G.; FRENCH, A.D., *Carbohydr. Res.*, 1995, **276**, 219.
[20] GIESEN, D.J.; CRAMER, C.J.; TRUHLAR, D.G., *J. Phys. Chem.*, 1995, **99**, 7137.
[21] GIESEN, D.J.; STORER, J.W.; CRAMER, C.J.; TRUHLAR, D.G., *J. Am. Chem. Soc.*, 1995, **117**, 1057.
[22] DEWAR, M.J.S.; ZOEBISCH, E.G.; HEALY, E.F.; STEWART, J.J.P., *J. Am. Chem. Soc.*, 1985, **107**, 3902.
[23] DEWAR, M.J.S.; ZOEBISCH, E.G., *J. Mol. Struct. (Theochem)*, 1988, **180**, 1.
[24] DEWAR, M.J.S.; YATE-CHING, Y., *Inorg. Chem.*, 1990, **29**, 3881.
[25] STEWART, J.J.P., *J. Comp. Chem.*, 1989, **10**, 221.
[26] HOIJTINK, G.J.; DE BOER, E.; VAN DER MEIJ, P.H.; WEIJLAND, W.P., *Recl. Trav. Chim. Pays-Bas*, 1956, **75**, 487.
[27] PERADEJORDI, F., *Cahiers Phys.*, 1963, **17**, 343.
[28] JANO, I., *Compt. Rend. Acad. Sci. Paris*, 1965, **261**, 103.
[29] KLOPMAN, G., *Chem. Phys. Lett.*, 1967, **1**, 200.
[30] TAPIA, O., In *Quantum Theory of Chemical Reactions*; Daudel, R., Pullman, A., Salem, L. and Viellard, A., Eds.; Reidel: Dordrecht, 1980, **2**, 25.
[31] CONSTANCIEL, R.; CONTRERAS, R., *Theor. Chim. Acta*, 1984, **65**, 1.
[32] CONTRERAS, R.; AIZMAN, A., *Int. J. Quant. Chem.*, 1985, **27**, 293.
[33] KOZAKI, T.; MORIHASHI, M.; KIKUCHI, O., *J. Am. Chem. Soc.*, 1989, **111**, 1547.
[34] TUCKER, S.C.; TRUHLAR, D.G., *Chem. Phys. Lett.*, 1989, **157**, 164.
[35] STILL, W.C.; TEMPCZYK, A.; HAWLEY, R.C.; HENDRICKSON, T., *J. Am. Chem. Soc.*, 1990, **112**, 6127.
[36] KING, P.M., In *Computer Simulation of Biomolecular Systems*; van Gunsteren, W.F., Weinger, P.K. and Wilkinson, A.J., Eds.; ESCOM: Leiden, 1993, **2**, 267.
[37] KIKUCHI, O.; MATSUOKA, T.; SAWAHATA, H.; TAKAHASHI, O., *J. Mol. Struct. (Theochem)*, 1994, **305**, 79.
[38] STORER, J.W.; GIESEN, D.J.; CRAMER, C.J.; TRUHLAR, D.G., *J. Comput.-Aid. Mol. Des.*, 1995, **9**, 87.
[39] MULLIKEN, R.S., *J. Chem. Phys.*, 1955, **23**, 1833.
[40] SINGH, U.C.; KOLLMAN, P.A., *J. Comp. Chem.*, 1984, **5**, 129.
[41] BESLER, B.H.; MERZ, K.M.; KOLLMAN, P.A., *J. Comp. Chem.*, 1990, **11**, 431.
[42] MERZ, K.M., *J. Comp. Chem.*, 1992, **13**, 749.
[43] CORNELL, W.D.; CIEPLAK, P.; BAYLY, C.I.; KOLLMAN, P.A., *J. Am. Chem. Soc.*, 1993, **115**, 9620.
[44] DEWAR, M.J.S.; THIEL, W., *J. Am. Chem. Soc.*, 1977, **99**, 4899.
[45] THIEL, W.; VOITYUK, A.A., *Int. J. Quant. Chem.*, 1992, **44**, 807.
[46] THIEL, W.; VOITYUK, A.A., *Theor. Chim. Acta*, 1992, **81**, 391.
[47] KOLB, M.; THIEL, W., *J. Comp. Chem.*, 1993, **14**, 775.
[48] SCHAEFER, M.; FROEMMEL, C., *J. Mol. Biol.*, 1990, **216**, 1045.
[49] LEE, B.; RICHARDS, F.M., *J. Mol. Biol.*, 1971, **55**, 379.
[50] ABRAHAM, M.H.; GRELLIER, P.L.; PRIOR, D.V.; DUCE, P.P.; MORRIS, J.J.; TAYLOR, P., *J. Chem. Soc., Perkin Trans.*, 1989, **2**, 699.
[51] ABRAHAM, M.H., *Chem. Soc. Rev.*, 1993, 73.
[52] ABRAHAM, M.H., In *Quantitative Treatments of Solute/Solvent Interactions*; Politzer, P. and Murray, J.S., Eds.; Elsevier: Amsterdam, 1994, 83.
[53] CRAMER, C.J.; TRUHLAR, D.G., *J. Am. Chem. Soc.*, 1991, **113**, 8552 and 9901(E).
[54] CRAMER, C.J.; TRUHLAR, D.G., *J. Am. Chem. Soc.*, 1993, **115**, 8810.
[55] CONTRERAS, J.G.; ALDERETE, J.B., *J. Mol. Struct. (Theochem)*, 1994, **309**, 137.
[56] CRAMER, C.J.; TRUHLAR, D.G., *J. Am. Chem. Soc.*, 1993, **115**, 5745.
[57] YANG, B.; WRIGHT, J.; ELDEFRAWI, M.E.; POU, S.; MACKERELL, A.D., *J. Am. Chem. Soc.*, 1994, **116**, 8722.
[58] RAO, B.G.; KIM, E.E.; MURCKO, M.A., *J. Comput.-Aid. Mol. Des.*, 1996, **10**, 23.
[59] URBAN, J.J.; CRAMER, C.J.; FAMINI, G.R., *J. Am. Chem. Soc.*, 1992, **114**, 8226.
[60] BARROWS, S.E.; CRAMER, C.J.; TRUHLAR, D.G.; WEBER, E.J.; ELOVITZ, M.S., *Environ. Sci. Technol.*, 1996, **30**, 3028.

[61] CHAMBERS, C.C.; ARCHIBONG, E.F.; JABALAMELI, A.; SULLIVAN, R.H.; GIESEN, D.J.; CRAMER, C.J.; TRUHLAR, D.G., *J. Mol. Struct. (Theochem)*, in press.
[62] CRAMER, C.J.; TRUHLAR, D.G., *J. Am. Chem. Soc.*, 1994, **116**, 3892.
[63] MCKEE, M.L., *J. Phys. Chem.*, 1993, **97**, 13608.
[64] SEVERANCE, D.L.; JORGENSEN, W.L., In *Structure and Reactivity in Aqueous Solution*; Cramer, C.J. and Truhlar, D.G., Eds.; American Chemical Society: Washington, DC, 1994, **568**, 243.
[65] ANGYAL, S.J., *Aust. J. Chem.*, 1968, **21**, 2737.
[66] HA, S.N.; GIAMMONA, A.; FIELD, M.; BRADY, J.W., *Carbohydr. Res.*, 1988, **180**, 207.
[67] BRADY, J.W., *J. Am. Chem. Soc.*, 1989, **111**, 5155.
[68] KROON-BATENBURG, L.M.J.; KROON, J., *Biopolymers*, 1990, **29**, 1243.
[69] VAN EIJCK, B.P.; KROON-BATENBURG, L.M. J.; KROON, J., *J. Mol. Struct.*, 1990, **237**, 315.
[70] HA, S.; GAO, J.; TIDOR, B.; BRADY, J.W.; KARPLUS, M., *J. Am. Chem. Soc.*, 1991, **113**, 1553.
[71] ZHBANKOV, R.G., *J. Mol. Struct.*, 1992, **275**, 645.
[72] POLAVARAPU, P.L.; EWIG, C.S., *J. Comp. Chem.*, 1992, **13**, 1255.
[73] VAN EIJCK, B.P.; HOOFT, R.W.W.; KROON, J., *J. Phys. Chem.*, 1993, **97**, 12093.
[74] GLENNON, T.M.; ZHENG, Y.J.; LE GRAND, S.M.; SHUTZBERG, B.A.; MERZ, K.M., JR., *J. Comp. Chem.*, 1994, **15**, 1019.
[75] DOWD, M.K.; FRENCH, A.D.; REILLY, P.J., *Carbohydr. Res.*, 1994, 264, 1.
[76] ZUCCARELLO, F.; BUEMI, G., *Carbohydr. Res.*, 1995, **273**, 129.
[77] HEHRE, W.J.; RADOM, L.; SCHLEYER, P.V.R.; POPLE, J.A., *Ab Initio Molecular Orbital Theory*; Wiley: New York, 1986.
[78] BARROWS, S.E.; STORER, J.W.; CRAMER, C.J.; TRUHLAR, D.G.; FRENCH, A.D., *J. Comp. Chem.*, in press.
[79] ANGYAL, S.J., *Angew. Chem., Int. Ed. Engl.*, 1969, **8**, 157.
[80] CRAMER, C.J.; TRUHLAR, D.G.; FRENCH, A.D., *Carbohydr. Res.*, 1997, **298**, 1.
[81] KIRKWOOD, J.G., *J. Chem. Phys.*, 1934, **2**, 351.
[82] ONSAGER, L., *J. Am. Chem. Soc.*, 1936, **58**, 1486.
[83] MÍCOVÍC, L.D.; ŽIGMAN, V., *J. Chem. Soc. Perkin Trans. II*, 1985, 625.
[84] DENBIGH, K., *The Principles of Chemical Equilibrium*, 4th ed., Cambridge University Press: London, 1981, 256–257.
[85] BEN-NAIM, A., *Statistical Thermodynamics for Chemists and Biochemists*, Plenum: New York, 1992, 421.
[86] GIESEN, D.J.; CHAMBERS, C.C.; HAWKINS, G.D.; CRAMER, C.J.; TRUHLAR, D.G., In *Computational Thermochemistry: Prediction and Estimation of Molecular Thermodynamics*; Irikura, K. and Frurip, D.J., Eds.; American Chemical Society: Washington, DC, in press.
[87] LOMBARDO, F.; BLAKE, J.F.; CURATOLO, W.J., *J. Med. Chem.*, 1996, **39**, 4750.
[88] TROHALAKI, S.; PACHTER, R., In *Abstracts of the 211th National Meeting of the American Chemical Society*; American Chemical Society: Washington, DC, 1996, COMP 60.
[89] RIBADENEIRA, M.D.; AUNGST, B.J.; EYERMANN, C.J.; HUANG, S.-M., *Pharm. Res.*, 1996, **13**, 227.
[90] GIESEN, D.J.; CHAMBERS, C.C.; CRAMER, C.J.; TRUHLAR, D.G., *J. Phys. Chem.*, in press.
[91] REYNOLDS, C.H., *J. Chem. Inf. Comput. Sci.*, 1995, **35**, 738.
[92] LEO, A.J., Masterfile database (1994) from MedChem Software.
[93] VAES, W.H.J.; URRESTARAZU RAMOS, E.; HAMWIJK, C.; VAN HOLSTEIJN, I.; BLAAUBOER, B.J.; SEINEN, W.; VERHAAR, H.J.M; HERMENS, J.L.M., *Chem. Res. Toxicol.*, 1997, **10**, 1067.
[94] WOHLFARTH, C., In *CRC Handbook of Chemistry and Physics*, 76th ed.; Lide, D.R., Ed.; CRC Press: Boca Raton, FL, 1995, 6–159ff.
[95] GONZALEZ-LAFONT, A.; TRUONG, T.N.; TRUHLAR, D.G., *J. Phys. Chem.*, 1991, **95**, 4618.

[96] LIU, Y.-P.; LU, D.-H.; GONZALEZ-LAFONT, A.; TRUHLAR, D.G.; GARRETT, B.C., *J. Am. Chem. Soc.*, 1993, **115**, 7806.
[97] BASH, P.; HO, L.L.; MACKERELL, A.D.; LEVINE, D.; HALLSTROM, P., *Proc. Natl. Acad. Sci., USA*, 1996, **93**, 3698.

CELL-BASED METHODS FOR SAMPLING IN HIGH-DIMENSIONAL SPACES

JASON A. RUSH*

Abstract. We regard the compounds in a combinatorial library of potential drugs as points in a Euclidean space of many dimensions, where the coordinates of a point represent properties used to characterize the compound it represents. By decomposing the space into certain advantageously selected Voronoi cells (not by the standard decomposition into hypercubes), and by choosing within each cell (e.g., for closer scrutiny, synthesis, etc.) a point near its center, one obtains conveniently small subsets that are highly representative of the larger library.

Introduction. It is a trivial exercise to propose so large a combinatorial library of potential drugs that a single molecule of each constituent would exhaust the mass of the known universe. From a more practical perspective, the library may be so large that one cannot afford to assay all elements. Therefore we want assurance that a sublibrary of tractable size is, in some sense, as representative as possible of the larger library. Suppose each compound is characterized by an n-tuple of real numbers, $(x_1, ..., x_n)$. These coordinates might quantify any of a number of properties of the compounds, for example

$\log P$,
dipole moment,
molecular weight,
surface area,
HOMO-LUMO-gap,

or quantities derived from these. The quantity $\log P$ is a measure of the difference in affinity of the compound for aqueous versus lipid solvents. Solubility in water is necessary for a drug to be available in body tissue, which is mostly water, but excessive lipophobicity interferes with transport across cell membranes. HOMO-LUMO gap is the distance between the highest occupied and the lowest unoccupied molecular orbitals. Pearlman [4] points out certain deficiencies with the above "traditional" descriptors. From our perspective, their chief deficiency turns out to be that there are not enough of them. Young et al. [5] also mention structural parameters such as

spacing of binding points,

which, along with certain graph-theoretic characterizations (like the presence or absence of specific rings or chains) adds quite a few more possible coordinates. Pearlman also introduces what he calls

BCUT values,

*Department of Mathematics, University of Washington, Seattle, WA 98195, USA.
fax: (206) 545-0847
phone: (206) 547-9952
email: jar@math.washington.edu

which are six eigenvalues of certain matrices whose on-diagonal information concerns

atomic charges
atomic polarizabilities, and
H-bond abilities,

and whose off-diagonal entries are of smaller magnitude and relate to the presence or absence of bonds between the atoms of the molecule.

The precise choice of descriptors used is not our main concern here, but I should mention desirable properties for a good set of descriptors. First of all, it would be nice if they were independent. Pearlman justifiably laments that the traditional ones are not. Second of all, it is desirable that biological activity be a continuous function of position in the n-dimensional parameter space, and that the coordinates have been so scaled that moving a unit distance in any direction should lead to the same change in biological activity. Third, it might be hoped that points far apart from one another have little in common as far as biological activity is concerned; however, this global condition seems too stringent. Indeed, there are plenty of dissimilar drugs with similar actions.

One may have only a poor notion of what the right scale factors are for the descriptors one has chosen, i.e., how the descriptors ought to be weighted. And choosing a set of descriptors that are both independent and chemically relevant is very difficult. These are serious problems. However, they are problems that are not specific to the cell-based strategy I suggest in this paper, but are generically endemic to any use of n-dimensional space to represent chemical compounds. Since the use of descriptors to classify compounds is here to stay, I make no apology for proceeding despite these problems. The method we describe allows the combinatorial chemist to design libraries of compounds that are far smaller yet (in an appropriate sense to be defined later) more diverse than would otherwise be possible.

This paper is an outgrowth of an insightful suggestion to me by Doehlert [2] that the cell-based method commonly used to partition n-space for the purpose of forming subsets (by selecting one point of the library from each hypercubic cell) seemed to him not to be ideally suited to the task, and that sphere-packing lattices might offer an advantage.

Notation and statement of the problem. Let U be an intractably large set of drugs from which we want to select a subset D for closer scrutiny, say for screening or synthesis. For the cardinalities of these sets (i.e., the number of elements in the sets) we write $|U|$ and $|D|$. How should one go about selecting the subset D of U? ("Diversity" is generally regarded as a property D should have; but this means different things to different people, and the extent to which the definition of diversity affects the nature of D has been insufficiently appreciated, particularly when the number n of dimensions is large.)

Let $U = \{u_1, ..., u_r\}$, $r = |U|$, and $D = \{d_1, ..., d_s\}$. Fix U and s. We use *dist* for the Euclidean distance between two points in our n-dimensional descriptor space.

Here are two common criteria for selecting members of D:

The spread criterion:
Choose $D \subset U$ so that the objective function $f(D) = \min_{\substack{i,j \\ i \neq j}} \text{dist}(d_i, d_j)$ is maximized. There are various alternatives to this particular objective function, for example one may decide to maximize $f(D) = \sum_{i=1}^{s} \min_{\substack{j \\ j \neq 1}} \text{dist}(d_i, j)$. But in the limiting case which will be our main concern, these have the same behavior, and we will not distinguish between them.

The coverage criterion:
Choose $D \subset U$ so that $f(D) = \max_{u_i \in U} \min_{d_j \in D} \text{dist}(u_i, d_j)$ is minimized. An alternative, and for our purposes of comparison, equally good (or poor) choice of the coverage criterion is the minimization of $f(D) = \sum_{u_i \in U} \min_{d_j \in D} \text{dist}(u_i, d_j)$.

These criteria, I believe, are less suitable than the fairly obscure *quantization criterion*, which unfortunately seems not to be used in the pharmaceutical field: Define $C_i = C(d_i) = \{u_j | \text{dist}(d_i, u_j) < \text{dist}(d_k, u_j) \text{ for all } k \neq i\}$. Then $d_1 \in C_1, ..., d_s \in C_s$. Also, the C_i partition, or tessellate U, aside from negligible boundary effects. That is to say, except for a small number of points of U that happen to be equidistant from two or more points of D, each point of U belongs to exactly one of the C_i. Choose $D \subset U$ so that $f(D) = \sum_{d_i \in D} \sum_{u_j \in C_i} \text{dist}^2(d_i, u_j)$ is minimized.

Regardless of the objective function one uses, finding its true global maximum may be impractical because it may be too expensive to evaluate the objective function (i.e., assay the potential drug) for all elements of U. Indeed, U may be so large that even enumerating each element in it may be unfeasible.

Notions from the geometry of numbers. Let Z^n denote the points of Euclidean n-space R^n whose coordinates all are integers. A lattice in R^n is a nonsingular linear transformation of Z^n. Let $\Lambda \subset R^n$ be a lattice, and let $x \in \Lambda$. The Voronoi cell (sometimes called the Dirichlet region; see [3], page 169) around x is $V(x) = \{y \in R^n | dist(x, y) \leq dist(w, y) \text{ for all } w \in \Lambda\}$. Voronoi cells around the lattice points provide a partition, or tiling, of R^n into convex, centrally symmetric polytopes.

Limiting case. The advantage of the quantization criterion over its two competitors becomes most apparent when moving to the limiting case $U = R^n$, $D = \Lambda$. Whereas we previously fixed s, we now fix $\det\Lambda$, the volume of a Voronoi cell. (In the literature, the determinant of a lattice is sometimes taken to mean not the volume of a Voronoi cell, but instead the square of that volume, so it is important to take note of the author's convention.) Actually s is analogous to $1/\det\Lambda$, the number of points of Λ per unit volume of space in R^n.

The spread, coverage, and quantization criteria assume these respective forms:

Continuous analog of the spread criterion

Among all lattices Λ in R^n having $\det\Lambda = 1$, find Λ so that the nearest face of $V(O)$ is as far as possible from the origin O . This is a famous classical problem in the geometry of numbers, namely, the problem of closest lattice-packing of spheres in R^n. It can be stated in this way: How can a lattice arrangement of non-overlapping spheres be chosen so that the largest possible fraction of R^n is occupied by them? That is, how can the density of the arrangement be maximized?

Continuous analog of the coverage criterion

Among all lattices Λ in R^n having $\det\Lambda = 1$, find Λ so that the farthest vertex of $V(0)$ is as close as possible to O. This is the problem of thinnest lattice covering of space by spheres, which is another famous classical problem in the geometry of numbers. Here the idea is to find a lattice arrangement of (necessarily overlapping) spheres that covers all of R^n, but as thinly as possible, i.e., with minimum density.

Continuous analog of the quantization criterion

Among all lattices Λ in R^n having $\det\Lambda = 1$, find Λ so that the second moment of $V(O)$ about its center, given by $\int\int \cdots \int_{V(0)} (x_1^2 + \ldots + x_n^2) dx_1 \ldots dx_n$, is minimized. This is a well-known classical problem in information theory: It is the problem of optimal design of analog-to-digital converters. (See, for example, [1], Chapter 2, §3.) What is wanted in this case is a lattice with the property that the expected squared distance from a random point of R^n (thought of as an analog signal) to the nearest point of the lattice (its digital approximation) is as small as possible. Thus, one thinks of the set of all possible drugs U as the universe of all possible analog signals, and the desired subset D as the optimal set of digital approximations to these signals.

What is the drug selection problem, anyway? Let me return to the problem I posed originally. U is an intractably large set of drugs from which we want to select a subset D for closer scrutiny. What is desired is that D should be as representative as possible of U . That is what the quantization criterion accomplishes. Drug selection is formally the same as analog-to-digital conversion.

The right number of descriptors. In general, the spread, coverage, and quantization criteria lead to different sorts of subsets D of U. This seems to have been insufficiently appreciated due to our reliance upon lower dimensions for visualization. Indeed, in one and two dimensions, all three criteria lead to the same optimal lattices. In one dimension, the Voronoi cells are equal intervals. In two dimensions, the Voronoi cells are regular hexagons. In three dimensions, the spread criterion leads to the face-centered cubic lattice, whose Voronoi cells are rhombic dodecahedra. The coverage and quantization criteria lead to the body-centered cubic arrangement, whose Voronoi cells are truncated octahedra.

It is seldom the case (that is, it is the case for only exceptional values of n) that the optimal lattice for any of these criteria is known for sure; however, there are many n for which quite good packings, coverings, and quantizers exist. There are reasonably good candidates for optimal lattices in dimensions through $n = 24$ for all three criteria. Standard sources of information on sphere packing and the geometry of numbers, such as Gruber and Lekkerkerker [3] and Conway and Sloane [1] contain much that is relevant to this discussion, as well as many further references.

A surprising aspect of this is that there are certain specific numbers of dimensions (for example 8 and 24) in which it is so advantageous to work, that if it is at all possible, the number of descriptors should be increased or decreased so that exactly 8 or 24 are used. This has nothing to do with chemistry. Its just that by combinatorial coincidence, extremely good packings, coverings and quantizers happen to exist in those dimensions. In fact, it is not even necessary to accept that quantization is better than spread or coverage. In dimension 24, the same lattice – the Leech lattice – apparently optimizes with respect to all three criteria.

Exploitation of the theory. The way in which the foregoing theory should be applied depends on the size of U. If U is small enough that direct evaluation of the quantization objective function $f(D) = \sum_{d_i \in D} \sum_{u_j \in C_i} \mathrm{dist}^2(d_i, u_j)$, which we seek to minimize, is possible, then that should be done. That is, one need do no more than replace the spread or coverage objective function with the above quantization objective function.

A more interesting and subtle application of the theory is possible if U is intractably large, so that the potential drugs are quite thickly strewn throughout a bounded region P (usually there are explicit numerical upper and lower bounds on the parameters, so that the region is an n-dimensional box) of the parameter space. (Then the limiting assumption $U = R^n$ is a close approximation to reality in that region.) Suppose that P has volume Vol P, and that a subset D of size s is desired. By means of a dilation (scale factor) one arranges for a quantization lattice Λ of determinant $\det\Lambda = \frac{\mathrm{Vol}\,P}{s}$ to be superimposed over P. Then, to form D, we take one point of U that lies close to the center of each Voronoi cell of Λ. Approximately s Voronoi cells of Λ will have centers in P, so this leads to a D of about the right size s. (Due to boundary effects, the exact size of D cannot be specified in any convenient way, but in practice the author has always found it easy to come close enough by making small adjustments to the dilation.)

Lattice decoding. For the process described above to be carried out in real time, it is necessary that one be able to solve the *lattice decoding problem* swiftly. This is the problem of finding the closest point of a lattice to any given point of space. For a general lattice, there is no quick way of doing this. Fortunately though, there are many excellent quantizing lattices that have fast, slick decoding algorithms. Dimensions 8 and 24 are advantageous not only for the reasons stated previously, but also because they offer fast decoding algorithms.

Let me introduce just enough coding theory to allow us to understand the mechanics of an 8-dimensional example.

An $[n, k, d]$ code C is a k-dimensional subspace of $GF(2)^n$ such that any two points (called codewords) of C differ in at least d places.

For example, the rows of the following matrix form an [8,4,4] code called a Hamming code:

1	1	1	1	0	0	0	0
0	0	1	1	1	1	0	0
0	0	0	0	1	1	1	1
1	0	1	0	1	0	1	0
1	1	0	0	1	1	0	0
1	1	1	1	1	1	1	1
0	1	0	1	1	0	1	0
0	0	1	1	0	0	1	1
1	0	0	1	0	1	1	0
1	0	1	0	0	1	0	1
1	1	0	0	0	0	1	1
0	1	1	0	0	1	1	0
0	1	0	1	0	1	0	1
1	0	0	1	1	0	0	1
0	1	1	0	1	0	0	1
0	0	0	0	0	0	0	0

Let C be an $[n, k, d]$ code. $\Lambda(C)$, the Construction A lattice of C, is defined as the union of the 2^k cosets of $2Z^n$ by the codewords of C. We may write this briefly as $\Lambda(C) = 2Z^n + C$. If we take C to be the $[8, 4, 4]$ code described above, then $\Lambda(C)$ is called E_8, and is an excellent quantizer that can be decoded by the following algorithm. Actually the algorithm applies to all binary Construction A lattices, not just E_8.

Algorithm for finding the closest point of $\Lambda(C)$ to a given point of R^n

(1) Given $x = (x_1, ..., x_n) \in R^n$, choose $y \in 2Z^n$ so that $0 \leq x_i - y_i < 2$ for $i = 1, 2, ..., n$.

(2) Replace x with $x - y$.

(3) Let $I = \{i | 1 < x_i < 2, i = 1, 2, ..., n\}$. For $i \in I$, replace x_i with $1 - x_i$.

(4) Let w be the closest point of Z^n to x. (Then w will be an n-tuple of zeros and ones, as it turns out.)

(5) Find the closest codeword c of C to w. (Depending on the code, a fancy algorithm may be called for here. The decoding of codes, as opposed to lattices, is a well-developed theory in its own right.)

(6) For $i \in I$, change c_i to $2 - c_i$.

(7) The closest point of $\Lambda(C)$ to the original x is $y + c$.

The 24-dimensional quantizing lattice, the Leech lattice, is not a Construction A lattice, but it also can be decoded quickly. It offers the ability to reduce the size of a combinatorial sublibrary by orders of magnitude without compromising representativeness.

Acknowledgments. Thanks to David Doehlert, Eric Martin, Jeff Blaney, George Lauri, and Dora Schnur for helpful discussions. The manuscript gained much clarity from Donald Truhlar's suggestions.

REFERENCES

[1] J.H. Conway and N.J.A. Sloane, Sphere packings, lattices and groups, Springer-Verlag, New York, second edition, 1993.

[2] D.H. Doehlert, personal communication.

[3] P. Gruber and C.G. Lekkerkerker, Geometry of numbers, Elsevier, Amsterdam, 1987.

[4] R.S. Pearlman, Novel software tools for addressing chemical diversity, Network Science, http://www.awod.com/netsci/Issues/Jun96/feature1.html.

[5] S.S. Young, M. Farman and Andrew Rusinko III, Random versus rational: Which is better for general compound screening? Network Science, http://www.awod.com/netsci/Issues/Aug96/feature3.html.

A PRELIMINARY MULTIOBJECTIVE ANALYSIS OF THE CHEMOTHERAPEUTIC BENEFITS OF HAIRPIN-LINKED POLYAMIDES

WYNN L. WALKER*, DAVID S. GOODSELL†, RICHARD E. DICKERSON*, AND ELLIOT M. LANDAW*

Abstract. In this study we review a mathematical model for estimating the free energies of binding for γ-aminobutyric-acid-linked polyamides containing N-methylimidazole and N-methylpyrrole to five- and six-base-pair DNA sequences. We use the model to evaluate numerically several different conflicting design criteria, each characterizing the suitability of a polyamide as a chemotherapeutic agent, and we analyze the trade-offs existing between these criteria. This preliminary analysis presents several methodological and modeling problems in the area of multiobjective optimization. We introduce some concepts from multiobjective optimization and conclude by discussing the application of these concepts to solving these problems.

1. Introduction. Drugs that bind to nucleic acids, blocking transcription and replication, are important in the treatment of cancer and AIDS related diseases. Many of the available drugs show limited sequence specificity and bind to many sites in a typical genome, leading to harmful side effects. Recently, the search for new chemotherapeutic agents has shifted to molecules designed to target a given DNA sequence in a pathogenic organism or neoplastic cell.

Polyamide molecules (such as the pyrrole-amide containing molecules netropsin and distamycin, and their imidazole-amide containing synthetic derivatives, known as lexitropsins) can bind double-stranded DNA in a sequence-specific manner (1-7). Linking of two polyamides enhances the binding to DNA and two modes of DNA binding have been reported for linked polyamides, the mode of binding being dependent on the linker choice (1). In one mode the linker enables the polyamides to bind DNA in an extended conformation. In the second mode the linker adopts a "hairpin" conformation so that the two polyamides are positioned side by side in the minor groove of DNA, enabling each molecule to recognize its own strand of DNA. Dervan and coworkers (1) report that polyamides linked via γ-aminobutyric acid favor binding in this second mode. An example of a hairpin-linked polyamide containing a triimidazole lexitropsin, a distamycin and a carboxy-terminal tail is shown in Figure 1 (3).

In hairpin-linked polyamides each pyrrole or imidazole ring makes contact with a single base. In addition, the γ-aminobutyric acid linker interacts with a single flanking base pair, and the carboxy-terminal tail interacts with the other flanking base pair. The sequence specificity results from the

*Departments of Biomathematics and Molecular Biology Institute, University of California, Los Angeles, Los Angeles, CA 90024, USA.

†Department of Molecular Biology, The Scripps Research Institute, La Jolla, CA 92037, USA.

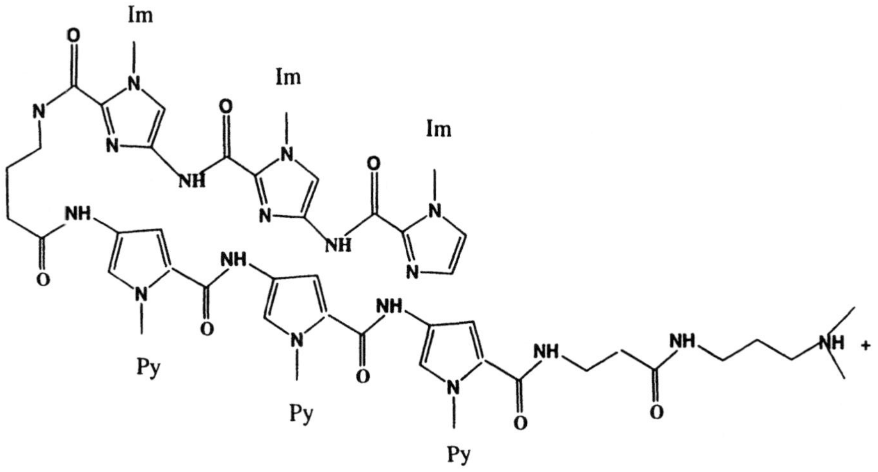

FIG. 1. *The molecular structure of a hairpin linked polyamide, ImImIm-γ-PyPyPy-β-Dp, an oligopeptide chain consisting of six peptide units. The peptide group in the upper right hand part of the molecule is the amino-terminal peptide group and the charged group in the bottom right is the carboxy-terminal tail.*

different hydrogen bonding capabilities of the pyrrole and imidazole rings as well as from the different interactions that the linker and tail have for base pairs containing adenine (A) and thymine (T) relative to base pairs containing guanine (G) and cytosine (C) (1-7). Empirical evidence suggests that imidazole binds preferentially to G, and pyrrole binds preferentially to A, C and T. The linker and tail preferentially bind A, T-containing base pairs.

Although pyrrole and imidazole show preferential binding to specific bases, they can also bind to a lesser degree to other bases. Therefore a polyamide designed to bind to a specific target DNA sequence may bind in a harmful manner to other host DNA sequences. In designing a polyamide for a given sequence, we can manipulate the strength of its binding for that sequence but must also take into account the strength of its harmful binding to nontarget host sequences. The ideal molecule would exhibit strong binding to a target sequence and little or no binding to nontarget sequences. However, as these two objectives cannot be optimized simultaneously, one must consider the design of a polyamide which provides the best compromise between the different criteria.

In this paper, we first review a linear regression model developed in an earlier study (8) for predicting the binding free energies of γ-aminobutyric acid hairpin-linked polyamides for five- and six-base-pair DNA sequences. We present a preliminary analysis of some of the trade-offs which exist among several different design criteria characterizing the suitability of a polyamide as a potential chemotherapeutic agent. The criteria studied include (1) the binding free energies of these polyamides for their target DNA sequences, (2) the fraction of the total amount of polyamide binding that is directed to the target sequence, (3) the ratio of the amount of polyamide binding to the target sequence relative to key host genome sequences, and (4) the fractional occupancy (saturation) of the available target sites. As a first step towards a unifying idea of how to rank the therapeutic values of these different criteria, we display and analyze the trade-offs that exist between different pairs of these criteria. This preliminary analysis raises additional important algorithmic and modeling issues in the area of multiobjective optimization. We conclude by defining some of these problems as well as possible approaches for their solution.

2. A mathematical model for the binding free energy of a polyamide to a DNA sequence. We considered a linear regression model for predicting the binding free energy of a polyamide to a DNA sequence. In doing so we assume that the free energy of binding of any given polyamide for a given DNA sequence is determined by the sum of the free energies of binding of each pyrrole-amide or imidazole-amide unit for the nearest base (and that there are no cross interactions between these units and other bases), the linker (γ-aminobutyric acid in this study) for its corresponding base pair, and the carboxy-terminal tail for its given base pair. We also assume that the free energies of linked three ring and linked four ring polyamides can be treated as similar additive sums of the individual base-ring interactions. This assumption may not hold for longer polyamides due to a slight mismatch between the length of a pyrrole (or imidazole)-amide repeat of the polyamide and the distance along the minor groove of DNA between two consecutive base pairs (9).

A complete model representing the above assumptions contains 12 free energy parameters in all: 4 of these are the free energies of interaction for each of the four bases with pyrrole, 4 are for the interactions of the four bases with imidazole, 2 are for the interactions of the aminobutyric acid linker with A, T-containing base pairs or G, C- containing base pairs, and 2 are for the interactions of the tail with A, T-containing base pairs or G, C-containing base pairs. However the full twelve parameter model is structurally unidentifiable from the available data, and we are forced to use a model of reduced dimensionality. The model we eventually settled on in (8) is given as follows:

$$\begin{aligned}\Delta G_{\text{bind}} = {} & \Delta G_{\text{end},AT} N_{\text{end},AT} + \Delta G_{\text{end},GC} N_{\text{end},GC} \\ & + \Delta G_{Im,ACT} N_{Im,ACT} + \Delta G_{Im,G} N_{Im,G} \\ & + \Delta G_{Py,AC} N_{Py,AC} + \Delta G_{Py,T} N_{Py,T} + \Delta G_{Py,G} N_{Py,G}.\end{aligned}$$

ΔG_{bind} is the dependent variable representing the free energy of interaction of a given polyamide with a given DNA sequence. $\Delta G_{\text{end},AT}$ and $\Delta G_{\text{end},GC}$ are parameters representing the free energies of binding of the γ-aminobutyric acid linker and the carboxy-terminal tail to AT or TA base pairs and GC or CG base pairs. (We assume that the energetics of binding is the same for both the hairpin linker and carboxy-terminal tail. Estimates for the difference between A, T- and G, C-containing base pair binding free energies using separate linker and tail parameters in an expanded version of this model were found to differ by only 0.3 kcal/mol.) $N_{\text{end},AT}$ ($N_{\text{end},GC}$) is the number of times that the first and/or the last base pairs in the DNA sequence (i.e. those adjacent to the tail and linker) is AT or TA (GC or CG). $\Delta G_{Im,G}$ and $\Delta G_{Im,ACT}$ are parameters for the binding free energies of imidazole (Im) rings respectively to G and A, C, and T bases. $\Delta G_{Py,AC}$, $\Delta G_{Py,T}$, and $\Delta G_{Py,G}$ are parameters for the binding free energies of pyrrole (Py) rings to A and C, for T, and to G respectively. $N_{Im,ACT}$, $N_{Im,G}$, $N_{Py,AC}$, $N_{Py,T}$, and $N_{Py,G}$ represent the number of times that an imidazole or pyrrole is nearest neighbor to the indicated base(s) in the corresponding subscript.

Several variants of this model with different parameterizations were initially considered. For each model, parameter estimates were determined based on an unweighted least squares fit to a data set containing 35 free energies of binding of different hairpin-linked polyamides for different DNA sequences using a linear regression program from BMDP statistical analysis software (10). We found that the above parameterization provided the best compromise out of all the models with regard to a good fit to the data as judged by the Akaike Information Criterion, AIC (11,12), the mean square error, MSE, and low standard errors (8). The AIC provides a measure of the model fit, relative to other candidate models, taking into account the number of adjustable parameters, P, the number of data points, N, and the residual sum of squares, RSS. Under Gaussian errors, $AIC = N \cdot ln(RSS) + 2P$. Also, $MSE = RSS/df$ where $df = N - P$ is the number of degrees of freedom. The parameter estimates and quality of model fit for the above model are summarized in Table 1. This model also demonstrated success in its predictive ability as determined through cross-validation experiments. These studies showed that the model is on average successful in predicting binding constants to within an order of magnitude and also in predicting less favorable free energies for sequences that experimentally show little or no binding of polyamide.

The model yields several physically meaningful interpretations. First of all, the highly negative value of $\Delta G_{\text{end},AT}$ and the slightly positive value for $\Delta G_{\text{end},GC}$ suggest a strong binding preference of the linker and tail for AT/TA base pair relative to GC/CG base pairs which is in accordance with experimentally observed data (3). This preference can be attributed to the unfavorable steric interactions that arise between atoms of the linker

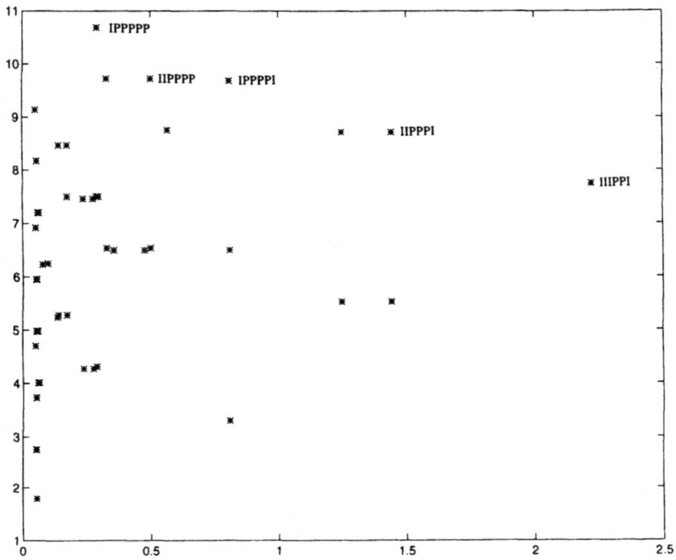

(A)

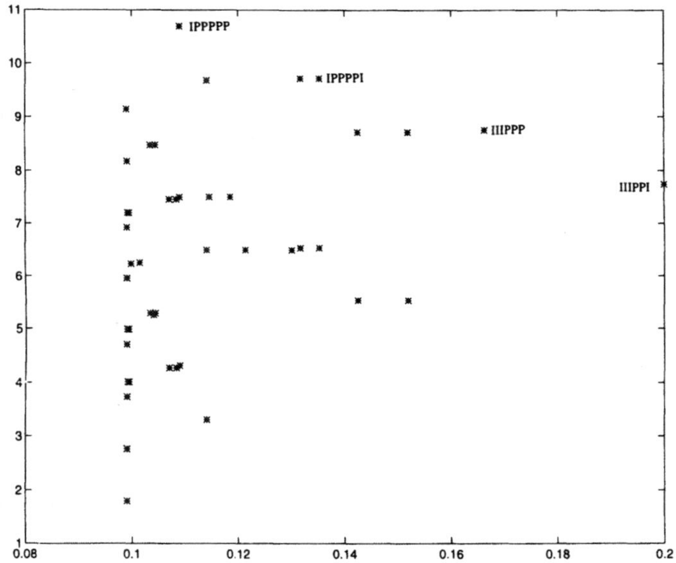

(B)

FIG. 2. *Plots of the negative of the binding free energy (kcal/mol), vertical axis, against* $\psi_{n,TATA}$*, horizontal axis, for the* 64 *polyamides at (A)* 50% *target sequence saturation, and (B)* 99% *target sequence saturation. The sets of nondominated polyamide solutions are indicated with labels, where I denotes an imidazole and P denotes a pyrrole. In the calculation of* ψ_n *we assume that the binding of each site is independent of the binding of the other sites and ignore the effects of binding interference due to overlapping sites.*

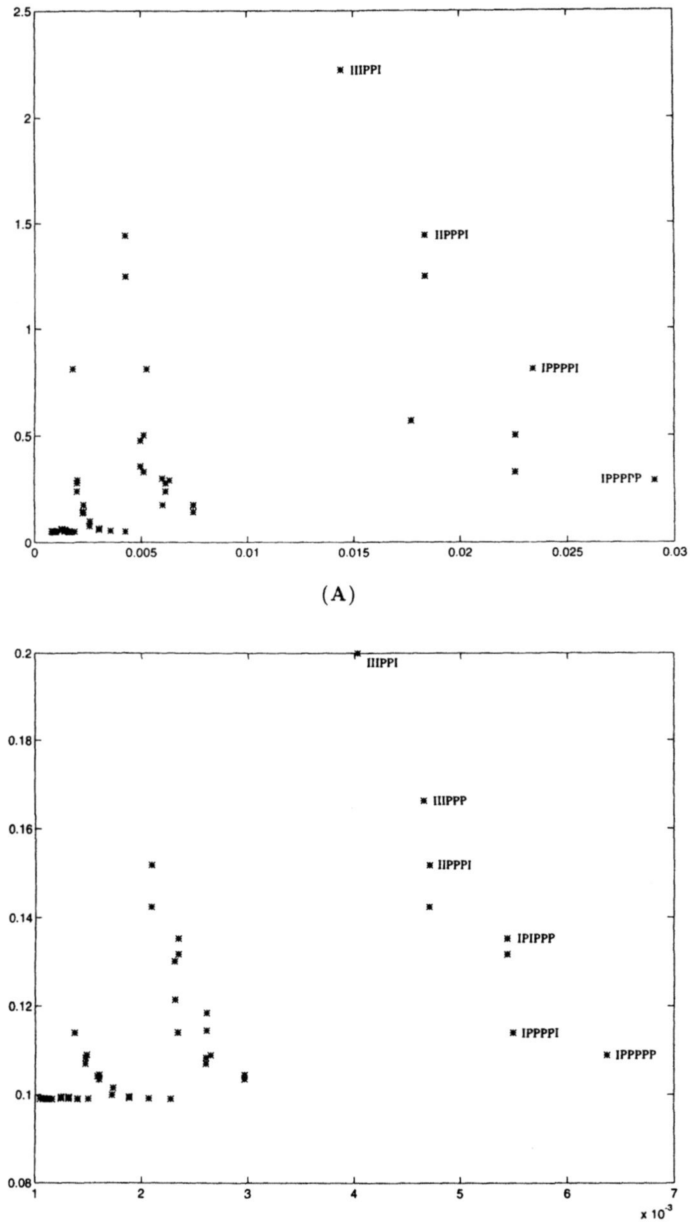

(A)

(B)

FIG. 3. *Plots of $\psi_{n,TATA}$, vertical axis, against ψ_n, horizontal axis, for the 64 polyamides at (A) 50% target sequence saturation, and (B) 99% target sequence saturation. The sets of nondominated solutions are indicated with labels. In the calculation of $\psi_{n,TATA}$ we assume that the binding of each site is independent of the binding of the other sites and ignore the effects of binding interference due to overlapping sites.*

TABLE 1

Summary of Parameter Estimates (kcal/mol) and Quality of Model Fit for Free Energy Models

Parameter Estimates and (Standard Errors)			Quality of Model Fit	
$\Delta G_{\text{end},GC}$	0.05	(0.77)	Residual Sum of Squares	19.47 (kcal/mol)^2
$\Delta G_{\text{end},AT}$	−2.14	(0.59)	Mean Square Error	0.70 (kcal/mol)^2
$\Delta G_{Im,ACT}$	0.42	(0.39)	degrees of freedom	35-7=28
$\Delta G_{Im,G}$	−1.20	(0.37)		
$\Delta G_{Py,AC}$	−0.54	(0.45)		
$\Delta G_{Py,T}$	−1.79	(0.36)		
$\Delta G_{Py,G}$	0.35	(0.42)		

or tail and the $N2$ amino group of guanine. The positive value for $\Delta G_{Py,G}$ suggests a free energy penalty for the recognition of a guanine by a pyrrole, consistent with a steric clash between the guanine $N2$ amino group and the pyrrole group. The positive value for $\Delta G_{Im,ACT}$ suggests that the imidazole-ACT mismatch is even more energetically unfavorable than the pyrrole-guanine mismatch. The relatively high free energy value predicted for these imidazole mismatches can be attributed to the burial of hydrogen bond acceptors on both the imidazole and the bases, losing water hydrogen bonds in the complex. The negative value of $\Delta G_{Im,G}$ indicates the favorable interaction between the imidazole and guanine, consistent with hydrogen bond formation between the imidazole nitrogen and the guanine $N2$ amino group. Finally the negative values of $\Delta G_{Py,AC}$ and $\Delta G_{Py,T}$ indicate favorable interactions of a pyrrole with the A, C, and T bases, consistent with their steric complementarity.

3. Prediction of polyamide sequence discriminatory ability. We applied the linear regression model to determine the free energies of binding for the 64 possible polyamides for the five-base-pair sequence $AGAAA$ (in this paper we only indicate the one strand of a double stranded DNA sequence written from 5′ to 3′). This sequence is an ideal target for the development of AIDS therapeutics: it is part of the polypurine tract of HIV-1, a sequence that is highly conserved among HIV-1 mutant strains and is not degraded by RNase H during reverse transcription (13-17). However, equally as important as the binding affinity of a drug for its target sequence is its ability to discriminate against other sequences. For instance, one might seek to minimize non-specific binding to the entire genome or to minimize binding to key sequences in the host genome such as the seven-base-pair TATA box consensus sequence TATA(A,T)A(A,T). The TATA box is a highly conserved regulatory sequence controlling the expression of human genes. Gene regulatory proteins known as transcription factors facilitate the transcription of DNA into RNA (i.e. the expression of genes) by binding to this sequence.

For each of these 64 six-ring compounds, we computed the binding affinities for each of the $4^5 = 1024$ possible five-base-pair sequences. Similarly, for each of the 256 eight-ring polyamides we computed the binding affinities for each of the $4^6 = 4096$ possible six-base-pair sequences.

With these free energy estimates, for a given polyamide one can estimate θ_i, the fractional occupancy or saturation of the available sites for the ith n-base-pair DNA sequence (i ranges from 1 to 4^n). This can be approximated mathematically by the following equation (4):

$$\theta_i = \frac{K_i[L]}{1 + K_i[L]}$$

where $[L]$ is the polyamide concentration, and K_i is its equilibrium association constant for binding with the ith sequence. K_i is related to the free energy ΔG_i, by the following equation: $K_i = \exp(-\Delta G_i/RT)$, where R and T are the gas constant and temperature respectively. Under the simplifying assumptions for this preliminary analysis that (1) each sequence appears with equal frequency in the genome, and (2) there is no significant interference or competitive binding at a site due to binding at neighboring overlapping sequences, the ratio ψ_n of polyamide binding to its intended n-base-pair target site, relative to all possible n-base-pair sequences, may be approximated by:

$$\psi_n = \frac{\theta_1}{\sum_{i=1}^{4^n} \theta_i}$$

($i = 1$ corresponds to the target site). Similarly, the ratio, $\psi_{n,TATA}$, of polyamide binding to its intended n-base-pair target site relative to all possible n-base-pair sequences contained in the TATA box consensus sequence may be approximated by

$$\psi_{n,TATA} = \frac{\theta_1}{\sum_{i_{TATA}} \theta_{i_{TATA}}}.$$

where i_{TATA} indexes the n-base-pair sequences contained in the TATA box consensus sequence. Thus $\psi_{n,TATA}$ is a measure of the ratio of binding to the target sequence relative to these TATA box sequences. A large value of $\psi_{n,TATA}$ means more specific binding to the target sequence relative to the TATA box sequences.

4. An analysis of the trade-offs existing between pairs of design criteria. With numerical measures of the different design criteria, the negative of the binding free energy to a DNA sequence ($-\Delta G_{bind}$), the percent saturation of the target sequence, (θ_1), the fraction of polyamide binding the target sequence, ψ_n, and the proportion of polyamide binding the target sequence relative to the TATA box sequences, $\psi_{n,TATA}$, we next analyze the suitability of different polyamide designs for the target sequence. Since there is no polyamide which simultaneously maximizes the objective functions $f_1, ..., f_k$ (the functions which represent the numerical measures of the k criteria), and we do not yet know the relative medical importance of the criteria with respect to each other, we generate a set of "nondominated solutions". These solutions can be thought of as the set of polyamides which summarize all compromises among the conflicting objectives. Mathematically stated, a polyamide design denoted by $x^* \in X$ (X is the design space which is the set of the $2^6 = 64$ six-ring polyamide designs) is a nondominated solution to the k-criteria multiobjective optimization problem if and only if there is no vector $x \in X$ with the characteristics

$$f_j(x) \geq f_j(x^*) \text{ for all } j \in \{1, ..., k\}, \text{ and}$$
$$f_j(x) > f_j(x^*) \text{ for at least one } j \in \{1, ..., k\}.$$

For ease of exposition, we look at $k = 2$ and display the set of points whose coordinates are given by $(f_1(x), f_2(x))$ for each $x \in X$ for the following two pairs of criteria: (1) $\psi_{n,TATA}$ and free energy, and (2) ψ_n and $\psi_{n,TATA}$. The points in the set of nondominated solutions are indicated with polyamide labels. We then present some observations regarding the relationship that exists between $\psi_{n,TATA}$ and θ_1, as well as between ψ_n and the polyamide length.

Free Energy and $\psi_{n,TATA}$: Figures 2A and 2B are plots of $-\Delta G_{bind}$ to the target sequence against $\psi_{n,TATA}$ for the 64 polyamides. Figure 2A represents conditions when half of the target sequence binding sites are occupied (i.e. 50% saturation); Figure 2B represents conditions for 99% saturation. The set of nondominated polyamides are indicated with labels in Figures 2A and 2B. From these plots, one can see as expected that for the nondominated solution sets the affinity of the polyamide for the target sequence is inversely related to the fraction of polyamide that binds the target sequence. One can also see that the distribution of polyamides in the nondominated set differs between Figures 2A and 2B, as do the percent saturations of the target sequence. This suggests that the polyamide providing the best compromise with regard to these two criteria may depend on the level of saturation that one wishes to achieve.

$\psi_{n,TATA}$ and ψ_n: Figures 3A and 3B are plots (at 50% and 99% target sequence saturation respectively) of $\psi_{n,TATA}$ against ψ_n for the 64 polyamides. These plots once again show the expected inverse relationship between ψ_n and $\psi_{n,TATA}$ for the nondominated polyamides, and the set of nondominated polyamides depends on the target sequence saturation level. A comparison of Figures 2A to 3A and of Figures 2B to 3B also shows a dependence of the nondominated solution set on the pair of criteria being optimized.

ψ_n and θ_1: For polyamide concentrations corresponding to a 50% and a 99% saturation of target sequences, ψ_n ranges from 0.014 to 0.029 and from 0.004 to 0.006 respectively in the nondominated sets. Therefore, ψ_n and θ_1 appear to be inversely related. A similar inverse relationship exists between $\psi_{n,TATA}$ and θ_1 ($\psi_{n,TATA}$ ranges from 0.35 to 2.2 at a 50% saturation of the target sequences and from 0.114 to 0.166 at a 99% saturation of target sequences).

Dependence of ψ_n on the Polyamide Length: Finally, the model calculations show a dependence of ψ_n on the polyamide length (i.e. the number of rings contained in the polyamide). For example, for a 50% saturation of the target sites, while the percentages of polyamide reaching the target site for the nondominated sets of eight-ring polyamides (which bind 5 base pair DNA sequences) range between 0.014 and 0.029, the corresponding percentages for the nondominated set of eight-ring polyamides (which bind 6 base pair DNA sequences) range between 0.006 and 0.014. The smaller percentages for the eight-ring polyamides demonstrate the counterintuitive idea that the percentage of molecules reaching the target site may decrease as the polyamide length increases. This is contrary to the usual expectation of enhanced specificity of molecules which cover a longer DNA sequence. However, the result for this model system can be accounted for by noting that there are approximately four times more six-base-pair sequences than five-base-pair sequences, and the intrinsic discriminatory abilities of the rings are not strong enough to overcome the increase in the number of sequences recognized. As a consequence, more nontarget sequences can be recognized by the longer polyamide than by the shorter polyamide.

5. Conclusions. In conclusion, these mathematical modeling studies have demonstrated that there are complex trade-offs between several different criteria which one might wish to optimize in the design of a chemotherapeutic agent. We have found that the optimal choices for polyamide design are quite sensitive to the choice of criteria to be optimized. Because of such a sensitivity, before one can effectively evaluate the optimality of polyamide designs we must address how to balance the dose of drug (which is directly related to the binding free energy and degree of desired saturation) against the lack of specificity of the polyamide.

Furthermore, more mathematical modeling and optimization issues are arising as we further investigate the biological issues relevant to the application of these polyamides as chemotherapeutic agents. For example, these studies are based on the assumption that each of the 4^n n-base-pair DNA sequences appears with equal frequency in the genome. Preliminary analysis shows that an over- or under-representation of the target sequence relative to the other possible sequences may have a significant effect on the values of both ψ_n and $\psi_{n,TATA}$. Likewise, the assumption of non-interference from binding at neighboring sites may be severely violated at high saturations.

With the appropriate mathematical descriptions of the criteria to be optimized, the need arises for the development of a methodology for rapidly generating and evaluating the set of nondominated solutions without exhaustively evaluating each criterion for all of the possible polyamide designs. With several criteria to optimize and a design space consisting of longer polyamides (for which there are many more possible polyamide designs) it becomes computationally burdensome to enumerate exhaustively all possible polyamide designs and isolate the nondominated solutions. However, the development of such a method is complicated by the fact that each nondominated solution set is not necessarily on the boundary of a convex set (see Figures 2A, 2B, 3A, and 3B). This nonconvexity precludes the application of simple methods for generating nondominated solutions, such as the method of objective weighting (18). Fortunately, the relatively simple system (a small design space of 64 polyamides and two criteria to optimize) is an ideal test system for the development and testing of algorithms for generating the nondominated solution set. Such algorithms could then be applied to the more complicated systems with a larger polyamide design space and more criteria to optimize. Given the nonconvexity of the nondominated solution set, we are testing the application of the reference point approach (19). In this method, aspiration values for each of the individual objectives are first specified and the nearest point (as determined by a specified norm) in the nondominated solution set is then computed. This procedure is iteratively repeated until enough nondominated alternatives have been generated for the given application.

Finally, the limitations of the discriminatory abilities of the pyrrole- and imidazole rings suggest a need for devising polyamide design alternatives with better discriminatory abilities than those of the existing pyrrole and imidazole-containing polyamides. This motivates the development of a computational algorithm to search for molecules with enhanced base-specific sequence discriminatory ability. For example, though the application of an algorithm that starts with a given polyamide as a lead compound and computationally performs a combinatorial search through various chemical modifications of this polyamide, it may be possible to find a molecule with base-reading units that more strongly discriminate among the given bases than do the imidazole and pyrrole rings.

6. Acknowledgments. We would like to thank Mary L. Kopka for all of her helpful comments.

This material is based upon work supported by a Fellowship from the Program in Mathematics and Molecular Biology at the University of California at Berkeley, which is supported by the National Science Foundation under Grant No. DMS-9406348. The Government has certain rights in this material. This work is also supported in part by NCI Grant No. CA-16042 and NIH Grant No. P01 GM48770. This is manuscript 10649-MB from the Scripps Research Institute.

REFERENCES

[1] Trauger, J.W., Baird, E.E., & Dervan, P.B., *Chemistry and Biology*, 3 (1996), 369–377.

[2] Parks, M.E., Baird, E.E., & Dervan, P.B., *J. Am. Chem. Soc.*, 118 (1996), 6147–6152.

[3] Swalley, S.E., Baird, E.E., & Dervan, P.B., J. Am. Chem. Soc., 118 (1996), 8198–8206.

[4] White, S., Baird, E.E., & Dervan, P.B., *Biochemistry*, 35 (1996), 12532–12537.

[5] Trauger, J.W., Baird, E.E., & Dervan, P.B., *Nature*, 382 (1996), 559–561.

[6] Cho, J., Parks, M.E., & Dervan, P.B., *Proc. Acad. Sci. U.S.A.*, 92 (1995), 10389–10392.

[7] Parks, M.E., Baird, E.E., & Dervan, P.B., *J. Am. Chem. Soc.*, 118 (1996), 6153–6159.

[8] Walker, W.L., Landaw, E.M., Dickerson, R.E., & Goodsell, D.S., *Proc. Natl. Acad. Sci. U.S.A.*, 94 (1997), 5634–5639

[9] Goodsell, D.S. & Dickerson, R.E., *J. Med. Chem.*, 29 (1986), 727–733.

[10] Dixon, W.J. (ed.), *BMDP Statistical Software Manual Volume 1*, University of California Press, Los Angeles (1990).

[11] Akaike, H., *IEEE Trans. Autom. Control model Identification*, AC19 (1974), 716–723.

[12] Landaw, E.M. & DiStefano, J.J. III., *Am. J. Physiol.*, 246 (Regulatory Integrative Comp. Physiol. 15) (1984), R665–R677.

[13] Gilboa, E., Mitra, S.W., Goff, S., & Baltimore, D., *Cell*, 18 (1979) 93–100.

[14] Rattray, A.J. & Champeux, J.J., *J. Virol.*, 61 (1987), 2843–2851.

[15] Resnick, R., Omer, C.A., & Faras, A.J., *J. Virol.*, 51 (1984), 813–821.

[16] Rattray, A.J. & Champeux, J.J., *J. Mol. Biol.*, 208 (1989), 445–456.

[17] Huber, H.E. & Richardson, C.C., *J. Biol. Chem.*, 265 (1990), 10565–10573.

[18] Eschenauer, H., Koski, J., & Osyczka, A., *Multicriteria Design Optimization*, Springer-Verlag, New York (1990).

[19] Wierzbicki, A, A Methodological Guide to Multiobjective Optimization. Proc. 9th Conference on Optimization Techniques, Springer-Verlag, New York, (ed.) Iracki, K., Malanowski, K., & Walukiewicz, S., 468–486.

USING STRUCTURAL INFORMATION FOR THE CREATIVE DESIGN OF MOLECULES

COLIN MCMARTIN* AND REGINE S. BOHACEK†

1. Introduction. Computer methods for molecular design have been steadily accumulating for several years. These methods use structural information from two major sources: the structures of known potent compounds and the structure of a target binding site. It is now possible to design compounds entirely using a *de novo* computer program [1], although it is more common for computer programs to be used to assist design by scientists. It is this latter process that will be discussed in this chapter.

A number of reports of successful computer assisted drug design are available [2–6]. In our experience, however, opportunities for using structural information are often missed. Even in projects where computer methods are applied, typically only a few compounds based on computer models are synthesized. The bulk of the compounds are made without any kind of assessment of their three dimensional properties.

We will argue that the lack of usage of computer models is only partly due to a need for improved computer algorithms. What is also needed is a new model or paradigm for the integration of computer methods into the drug design process.

2. Understanding the potency and specificity of drugs. Towards the end of last century, it was discovered that certain simple organic molecules have beneficial therapeutic properties. These compounds often work with exquisite specificity at very low concentrations. The list of targets for which a specific molecule can be found appears to be almost endless. It is also clear that small changes in molecular structure can sometimes have dramatic effects in specificity and potency. These molecules are often quite small, yet they operate selectively in a biological environment of staggering complexity. What is the scientific explanation for these remarkable properties?

For a number of years now, structural biology has been providing convincing experimental confirmation of one of the earliest hypotheses, the lock and key model of the pioneering chemist Emil Fischer [7]. Numerous X-ray studies of molecules interacting with a specific protein target have shown the molecule bound to a cavity in the protein. In all the cases that I am aware of where the molecule is of high potency, the spatial fit is almost perfect, and in addition there are a number of well-positioned hydrophobic and hydrogen bonding contacts.

*Thistlesoft, 302 Lindsley Drive, Morris Township, NJ 07960.
†ARIAD Pharmaceuticals, 26 Landsdowne St., Cambridge, MA 02139.

The hypothesis that interaction with specific binding sites is the key to understanding potency and hence selectivity has been quantitatively validated and empowered by calculations of the relative free energies of different ligands in the same binding site [8]. The method uses molecular mechanics force fields, derived independently of drug interaction studies, to carry out molecular dynamics simulations. The method of calculation is based on statistical perturbation theory that, in turn, is rigorously derived from classical thermodynamics and statistical mechanics. Excellent agreement with experimental binding affinities is often obtained.

While this is satisfying theoretically, the question now is: How can we apply this knowledge to the design of potent and selective drugs against new targets? Part of the answer to this question is that we need rapid and reliable methods for estimating the potency of compounds prior to synthesis. Simply satisfying this need, however, does not take account of the fact that the synthetic candidates must first be designed or discovered by some process. The next two sections will explore the design process and ways of facilitating it in more detail.

3. Drug design as a creative process. The design of drugs is at present a largely human endeavor. It could be argued that *de novo* design or *de novo* optimization by computer programs will eventually furnish 'ready to make' molecules that, once synthesized, will be found to have the potency, specificity and bioavailability required of an effective therapeutic agent. At present, this is far from being achieved (see below), although *de novo* methods can certainly provide inspirational starting points for optimization and modification prior to synthesis.

A major concern of those involved in drug design is that computer methods will act as a limiting filter that will interfere with the tried and tested methods of discovery and lead optimization. This section will describe drug design as a creative process and show how appropriate computational feed-back on proposed ideas can actually enhance creativity.

In the present context, creativity will be taken to mean a process in which: (a) multiple choices are available, (b) these choices are made in a skillful and original manner, and (c) a design is achieved that satisfies a set of well defined requirements.

It is not difficult to see that the range of choices for designing molecules is very large. Just how large has recently started to become apparent. It has been estimated that the number of molecules containing 30 atoms exceeds 10^{60} [2]. At the same time the number of compounds that can be designed to be complementary to a binding site of even modest size has been estimated using a powerful *de novo* design program to be around 10^{27} [1]. Thus there is an enormous wealth of choices and the number of reasonable solutions, although possibly 30 orders of magnitude smaller, easily exceeds our human grasp.

It is clear that designers of molecules, knowingly or otherwise, are working on a very broad canvas. In order to reach design specifications, knowledge and intuition are required. The successful medicinal chemist or computational drug design expert has a large amount of knowledge and experience which, at present, lies outside the scope of computer methods. Computational methods can, however, provide answers to questions involving very complex calculations or data searching operations that are otherwise completely inaccessible. What is needed is a partnership of these two skills bases.

To accomplish this in an optimal fashion, the designer should be able to interact freely with the computer. This can be achieved using an interface that allows critical queries to be effortlessly launched and rapidly answered. Computer generated information should be informative, easily interpreted, and almost as accessible as the user's own knowledge and experience. This will allow the designer to rapidly explore and refine ideas. In my experience such a process allows a wider range of ideas to be explored before compounds are synthesized. The process becomes more creative in terms of skill and originality by permitting larger changes in an initial lead structure or idea while staying on the design target.

4. Design strategies that use structural information. This section will identify general questions that computer modeling can answer. Available algorithms and programs will be discussed in the section following this one.

Design strategies are highly dependent on the available information. We will start by considering a worst case scenario and proceed to examine situations where progressively more information is available.

(a) Starting with a small number of low potency leads. In the majority of projects the structures of one or more active compounds will be known. Typically at the start these will not be very potent, perhaps around 10 μM. Often the compounds will be flexible. This represents the most difficult situation for design. If the aim is a 10 nM drug, it is likely that the final compound will differ significantly from the starting point and, yet, there is little or no information to indicate what changes need to be made. Nevertheless structural information is used in the search for more active compounds. Usually changes are made to parts of the structure while conserving other features as part of a search strategy. This phase of a project is also influenced by the outlook of the medicinal chemist. For some, the goal is simply to most rapidly discover an active compound. Others will be more open to the idea of searching a variety of modifications to understand the structure activity relationships. The approach will, of course, have a significant effect on the efficiency of modeling at later stages in the project. Although computer methods are difficult to use at this stage, it is possible that they could assist in the search process in two ways.

1. By assessing the 3-*D* match between new synthetic targets and parts of the structure that the designer would like to conserve. This could open up the possibility of changing the chemistry to facilitate ease of analogue design.

2. By providing 3-*D* models that show precisely how proposed synthetic structures differ from the starting structure and from each other.

In addition it seems possible that a computer program might be able to provide information on the most efficient choices to make in the search, although to my knowledge methods for doing this remain to be discovered.

A second strategy would be to design a focused combinatorial library to be able to rapidly find hits or explore the structure-activity relationships. This will frequently involve basic changes in the chemical structure of the lead compound in order to find a suitable combinatorial base template. Choosing the template and the side chains or monomers can be greatly assisted by computer modeling information. Ideally, the library will contain at least some 3-*D* analogues of the starting structure as well as many structures that are reasonably close to it.

(b) When potent active analogues are available. As a project progresses a wealth of structure activity data starts to accumulate. If an active compound is non-flexible it is easy to produce a geometrically precise 3-*D* model using molecular mechanics. Other flexible compounds can now be fitted to the model to see if a consensus model can be generated. If only flexible active compounds are available, it is possible to carry out a flexible search for conformers that overlap. This will sometimes produce a unique solution that can be taken as a 3-*D* model or it may produce a number of alternative models. A 3-*D* model of an active analogue can also sometimes be obtained by NMR studies of the analogue interacting with its target. This can be achieved even when the structure of the target has not been determined.

If a 3-*D* model of reasonably potent compounds is available, it is essential that computer modeling is integrated into the design process if the model is to be exploited fully. Simply looking at pictures of the model and designing compounds on a sheet of paper very rarely produces compounds that match the model. The questions that can be asked are:

1. How well does the design idea match the target (sterically and chemically)

2. What is the internal energy of the structure relative to its global minimum

3. What changes are indicated to improve the match or internal energy

If sufficient data are available, it should be possible to produce a potency model that will give an estimated potency. If the model is found to produce reasonable predictions ahead of synthesis, it will be of enormous value in the process of designing and selecting compounds for synthesis.

(c) When structural data is available for the binding site. Availability of a model of a binding site often generates considerable excitement in a project. All the information is available to design novel potent inhibitors, so the problem appears to be almost solved. In practice, this is hardly ever true and the information in binding site models is often not fully exploited. First it is necessary to establish that the model is reasonable for the types of compound being designed. This means that when lead compounds are docked and evaluated using molecular mechanics, one or more low energy binding modes can be found. Where this is not the case, flexibility can be introduced into the binding site. If this flexibility is supported by experimental data, e.g. differences have been observed in X-ray structures for different ligands in the binding site, it is reasonable to introduce such flexibility. Otherwise the introduction of flexibility may result in making the molecule too permissive so that inactive compounds may be modeled as active.

When a reasonable model of the binding site is available, computer modeling can assist in design in a number of ways:

1. Assessing how well design ideas fit the model (steric and chemical complementarity);
2. Estimating the potency prior to synthesis;
3. Designing focused combinatorial libraries;
4. *De novo* design of molecules that show structural and chemical complementarity, that dock at low energy, and that are assessed to be potent.

In practice, structural information on the binding site is rarely fully used in a project. Despite major investments in NMR and X-ray and numerous reports of success, in my experience in many projects the structural data only has a marginal impact. For a variety of reasons (and non-reasons), the tools that are available to assist drug design are not integrated fully into the design process. This also applies to active analogue (pharmacophore) modeling. I will propose solutions to this problem later.

5. Computer algorithms that use structural information. The number of programs that have been developed to assist drug design is very large. This section will describe basic algorithms with specific examples of programs. The omission of a program in no way reflects my partiality and we apologize to the writers of such programs. Where appropriate, the performance of our own programs QXP and Growmol is presented in more detail since we have first-hand experience with these programs.

(a) Making 3-D pharmacophore models. A number of effective methods for developing models from flexible active molecules are available [9–11]. These methods use conformational searching. The atoms or functional groups that are to be matched may be specified by the user or selected by the program [10,11]. My own program [QXP,11] uses a superposition force field. In this method atoms of similar chemical type but in different molecules experience an attractive potential. Superposition energy and internal molecular mechanics energies are then cominimized. The force field was validated and optimized by testing its ability to predict bioactive conformations of thermolysin inhibitors that are known for X-ray analysis [12].

(b) Design based on pharmacophore models. Some of the methods for making models described above also can be used for this purpose, except that now the model is kept fixed and a proposed design idea is fitted. I find the superposition force field very convenient for this purpose since the match to all atoms is optimized. With a suitable graphics interface it is possible to sit at the screen, rapidly modify a test structure and launch a minimization. Within seconds the result can be read in and examined visually. Information on the internal energy of the ligand is also useful. Rather than do this as a separate job (which requires separating the ligand from the pharmacophore, calculating its energy and then searching for the global minimum), all the procedures can be bundled in one application. Thus, launching a single job returns information on the geometric match as well as the energy cost. With this information it is possible to decide whether the compound is a reasonable synthetic target or requires further modification. Detailed applications of this method have been published [5–6].

(c) Using potency models based on active compounds. Potency models are typically grid maps that contain information about the contribution to potency of each atom of the molecule according to the atom type and the grid point it occupies. Examples of programs that use different algorithms to prepare the potency model include HASSL [13] and COMFA [14]. These methods have been shown to produce reasonable results in some cases and might be beneficial in a number of projects where structure activity data is available. It may be hard to tell in advance how well they will work for a given application and set of data. A possible solution to this problem may be to develop and automate these methods so they can effectively go on line at minimal user cost . This concept will be discussed further later.

(d) Design with knowledge of a binding site. Design in a binding site can be greatly facilitated using binding site surface maps to show where specific types of ligand atom should be placed. The program GRID [15] produces contour maps showing optimal positions for small functional groups calculated using a force field. We have developed a program that generates a Lee and Richards accessible surface and colors it for complementarity using an algorithm derived from a study of complementarity of packing in high resolution X-ray structures of proteins [16]. This surface shows with precision where ligand atoms should lie in order to be in contact with the binding site atoms. In our experience, when the surface is applied to the binding site found in X-ray structures of ligand complexes, the ligand is always found to show high levels of steric and chemical complementarity to the binding site. Although these surface models can provide a powerful guide for the design of compounds, it is nevertheless impossible to tell how well a design idea will work without, at the very least, energy minimization and evaluation of the proposed structure in the binding site.

Thus, binding site design requires evaluation of docking of known and test compounds. A number of docking methods have been published . For design applications the method should enable complete conformational searches of all test structures with full energy minimization in the binding site. It is also useful to be able to allow parts of the binding site to move during minimization. An early study of docking using BATCHMIN fulfills these requirements [17]. The procedure in QXP is also based on Monte Carlo searching with energy minimization in Cartesian space [9]. The QXP procedure has been further developed to increase speed and incorporate automatic searching for the global minimum energy of the free ligand as well as automatic calculation of relevant interaction energies.

This allows interactive design at the graphics terminal. The ligand structure is modified and a docking application launched with minimal user effort. The most rapid application returns a minimized structure along with critical energies including the internal ligand energy relative to its global minimum in a few seconds. Full docking searches take time ranging from minutes to up to three hours, depending on the size of the molecule, the number of search steps, and the power of the processor. Several applications to drug design using this program have been published [4–6]

(e) Potency estimation based on a binding site structure. A number of algorithms have been described [18–21]. Empirical scoring functions can, in principle, rapidly predict the potency of a ligand without any reference compounds [18,19]. Methods based on short molecular dynamics simulations and a semi-empirical approximation also calculate the potency of ligands, without the need for a reference compound [20]. Finally, thermodynamic perturbation methods can be applied to calculate differences between potency of a novel ligand and a close analogue [21]. If the potency of the analogue is known, the potency of the new compound can then be estimated. As with potency models based on active compounds, there is uncertainty in the user community about which, if any, methods will work in a given application. Solutions to this problem will be discussed in the next section.

It is also possible to generate molecules in a binding site using *de novo* methods [1]. These methods are discussed in another chapter of this book.

6. Integrating modeling methods into the design process. To effectively integrate computer methods we need to be aware of the perspective of medicinal chemists and their managers. One of the major concerns is that computer modeling will use up resources and divert the discovery process away from tried and tested, albeit very inefficient, methods. In contrast, the inventors of computer methods, naturally enough, believe that their methods will provide a hitherto-lacking focus that is worth any additional cost or inconvenience. A compromise solution that is sometimes tried is to introduce a small amount of modeling in a project as an experiment. This approach, with its manifest lack of commitment, is usually not very successful. Most of the compounds that are made are not modeled and, even although most of these are not potent, any successes will be taken as proof that modeling is not necessary, whereas failures of a small number of modeled compounds are taken to indicate that modeling is unreliable.

Our recent has experience has been that the conflict of interest does not arise if the computer methods are easy to use, and rapid, and are used initially only for questions that can be reliably answered by the computer but which cannot otherwise be answered by the user. These primary questions are structural. How well does a design idea match existing structures? How does it dock in a binding site? These questions are almost always in the mind of the chemist when design ideas are being proposed and it is natural to try to answer them if methods are readily available that give rapid and reliable results.

We have been developing both graphics and molecular mechanics programs with this goal in mind. Our experience in the last two to three years has been encouraging. It is usually found that the first design ideas do not have the desired 3-D structural characteristics. This produces an incentive to design additional compounds to obtain a better match. Our program also provides indications of features that may need to be changed. In some projects up to 50 molecules are designed to find one that meets the structural target well and is then synthesized.

This process provides molecules that meet primary design specifications, e.g. reasonable match to a pharmacophore with low internal energy or reasonable fit in a binding site with hydrogen bond and hydrophobic contacts. The proposed solutions could now be further examined using methods to estimate potency. Since it is often difficult to tell which, if any, methods will work, we propose that several methods are routinely and automatically applied so that no extra user effort is required. This data should then be examined when biological results are reviewed. If the potency parameters correlate with potency, the relevant models can then be introduced into the process of design and selection for synthesis. Computer experts can continue to refine and develop models that are not working well.

Integration might be further improved by putting modeling 'on line' in a project in parallel with the primary biological screens. When a structural model is available, all compounds synthesized should be automatically modeled as soon as their structure is registered and they are sent for biological testing. The modeling results can then go into a data-base alongside the potency results. This could be applied to molecules without any human effort, regardless of whether or not the molecules were initially modeled. Having modeling data available in conjunction with potency data for all compounds will generate a rational desire to design using modeling methods that are helpful, and avoiding those methods that are misleading.

7. Conclusions. This chapter is based on our current experience of how computer programs are used in drug design and on a vision of how they might be used. We have focused on the process of designing new molecules and have omitted extremely important aspects, such as database searching for new leads. Our conclusion is that computer methods can have an enormous impact on the design process that rarely reaches its full potential in daily practice. In the next few years we anticipate that this potential will be realized as methods are integrated with graphics interfaces to provide more ideal environments for creative design, and as the validity of accurate methods for estimating potency becomes established.

REFERENCES

[1] Bohacek, R.S. and McMartin, C., J. Am. Chem. Soc. (1994), 116:5560.
[2] Bohacek, R.S., McMartin, C., and Guida, W.C., Medicinal Research Reviews (1996), 16:1.
[3] Greer J., Erickson, J.J., Baldwin, J.J., and Varney, M.D., J. Med. Chem. (1994), 37:1035.
[4] Bohacek, R.S., de Lombaert, S., McMartin, C., Priestle, J., and Gruetter, M., J. Am. Chem. Soc. (1996), 118:8321.
[5] Ksander, G.M., de Jesus, R., Yuan, A., Ghai, R.D., Trapani, A., McMartin, C., and Bohacek, R.S., J. Med. Chem. (1997), 40:495.
[6] Ksander, G.M., de Jesus, R., Yuan, A., Ghai, R.D., McMartin, C., and Bohacek, R.S., J. Med. Chem. (1997), 40:506.
[7] Fischer, E., Ber. Dtsch. Chem. Ges. (1894), 27:2985.
[8] Merz, K.H. and Kollman, P.A., J. Am. Chem. Soc. (1989), 119:5649.
[9] McMartin, C. and Bohacek, R.S., J. Computer-aided Mol. Des. (1997), in press.
[10] Martin, Y., Bures, M.G., Danher, E.A., DeLazzer, J., Lico, I., and Pavlik, P.A., Computer-Aided Mol. Des. (1993), 7:83.
[11] Mayer, D., Naylor, C.B., Motoc, I., and Marshall, G.R., J. Computer-Aided Mol. Des. (1987), 1:3.
[12] McMartin, C. and Bohacek, R.S., J. Computer-Aided Mol. Des. (1995), 9:237.
[13] Doweyko, A.M., J. Med. Chem. (1988), 31:1396.
[14] Cramer III, R.D., Patterson, D.E., and Bunce, J.D., J. Am. Chem. Soc. (1988), 5959.
[15] Goodford, P., J. Med. Chem. (1985), 28:849.
[16] Bohacek, R.S. and McMartin, C., J. Med. Chem. (1992), 35:1671.
[17] Guida, W.C., Bohacek, R.S., and Erion, M.D., J. Comp. Chem. (1992), 13:214.
[18] Boehm, H.-J., J. Computer-Aided Mol. Des. (1994), 8:243.
[19] Head. R.D., Smythe, M.L., Oprea, T.L., Waller, C.L., Green, S.M., and Marshall,G.R., J. Am. Chem. Soc. (1996), 118:3959.
[20] Hansson, T. and Aqvist, J., Protein Engineering (1995), 8:1137.
[21] Kollman, P. Chem. Rev. (1993), 93:2395.

GROWMOL, A De novo COMPUTER PROGRAM, AND ITS APPLICATION TO THERMOLYSIN AND PEPSIN: RESULTS OF THE DESIGN AND SYNTHESIS OF A NOVEL INHIBITOR

REGINE BOHACEK*, COLIN MCMARTIN†, PETER GLUNZ‡, AND DANIEL H. RICH§

Abstract. The conceptual basis for structure-based drug design was formulated 100 years ago by Emil Fisher(1) . His "lock and key" hypothesis is a constantly recurring theme in modern drug design. Previously, knowledge of the "lock", i.e. the biochemical target, could only be inferred by the structures of a variety of "keys" (ligands) all of which fit the "lock". However, thanks to the advances in protein expression, X-ray crystallography and NMR, more and more often we now actually have the three dimensional structure of the biological target. And, thus, the new challenge is how to utilize this information to rapidly discover novel, potent molecules which will exquisitely fit the "lock".

A number of computational methods are emerging which use three dimensional structures to automatically design, *de novo*, molecules which fit into binding sites. We describe here the development and use of a computer program called GrowMol(2, 3), which generates organic structures that are both spatially and chemically complementary to the target binding site. By "growing" molecules an atom at a time to fill the various nooks and crannies of a binding site, GrowMol can generate structures with exquisite complementary to the host. At each step, the position and type of atom to be added are randomly selected using Boltzmann statistics to bias acceptance toward atoms that can form favorable interactions with the binding site. GrowMol was first tested with thermolysin. The program generated known inhibitors as well as large numbers of novel, diverse structures complementary to the thermolysin binding site. Recently, GrowMol was applied to the aspartic acid protease, pepsin, resulting in the discovery of a novel, low molecular weight inhibitor. (4)

Introduction. The dramatic increase in the number of crystal structures of biologically important molecules offers a unique opportunity for the design of novel drugs. In principle, the accurate three dimensional structure of a binding site provides all the information required for the design of high affinity drugs. One of the major challenges for computer aided drug design is the development of computational methods to exploit this structural data.

One of the most exciting and active areas of computational chemistry is the development of computer programs which automatically generate molecules into the three dimensional structure of a host binding site. These methods are able to suggest new ligands, designed *de novo*, which complement the binding site both spatially and chemically.

*ARIAD Pharmaceuticals, 26 Landsdowne St., Cambridge, MA 02139

†Thistlesoft, 302 Lindsley Drive, Morris Township, NJ 07960

‡The School of Pharmacy, University of Wisconsin-Madison, Madison, WI 53706

§The School of Pharmacy and the Department of Chemistry, University of Wisconsin-Madison, Madison, WI 53706

Since the early 1990's, a number of different strategies have been developed for creating novel molecules in binding sites(5, 6, 7). Several methods use large sets of molecular fragments that are docked into energetically favorable sites in the receptor. These fragments can subsequently be linked together to form molecules. (8) Another strategy is to flood the binding site with atoms or small fragments, optimizing their position using dynamics and then determine the best ways to connect these fragments to form molecules. (9, 10, 11, 12, 13, 14, 15) A third approach is to "grow" molecular structures into a binding site one atom or small fragment at a time. (5, 16) This is the approach used in our *de novo* program, GrowMol. (2)

By growing molecules an atom at a time to fill the various nooks and crannies of a binding site, GrowMol can generate a large variety of different structures with high degrees of complementarity to the host. At each step the position and type of atom to be added is randomly selected from a set of possible values consistent with internal bond lengths and bond angle requirements as well as the spatial and chemical properties of the binding site. The selection is achieved using Boltzmann statistics to bias the acceptance toward atoms which can form favorable interactions with the binding site. Rings are generated by connecting closely positioned nonbonded atoms. This procedure ensures generation of a highly diverse set of structures unbiased by knowledge of known guest ligands.

To identify structures most likely to bind well to the enzyme, the binding conformation of each grown structure is further optimized by energy minimization. Next the structures are evaluated and ranked using a scoring algorithm based on chemical complementarity. The scoring function was tested with a set of thermolysin inhibitors. Good correlation was found between the experimentally determined potency and that estimated using this algorithm.

A preliminary test for a *de novo* program is the generation of ligands already known experimentally to have high affinity for the target. The *de novo* generation of known ligands is a good test both for the program's structure generation and scoring algorithms. An indication of the difficulty of *de novo* ligand generation is that only a few of the existing programs have been reported to generate, *de novo*, ligands known to bind to the target. In order to generate known ligands, the building blocks used must be small enough or numerous enough so that when linked together they can form a wide range of different organic molecules. In addition, a *de novo* program must be able to do extensive sampling since the smaller the building blocks used to construct molecules, the larger the number of possible molecular structures. The scoring function which is used to drive the optimization of the structures must also be sufficiently accurate to be able to recognize some of the features which cause the binding of known potent ligands. GrowMol is one of the few *de novo* programs which includes known ligands in its output.

Method

There are three main steps in the generation of structures by GrowMol: a grid map is calculated for the binding site, the molecular structures are generated and finally, the structures are evaluated and ranked.

Binding site grid map. Calculation of the binding site grid map is based on earlier work in which the Lee and Richards accessible surface was used as a graphical aid for viewing protein binding sites and evaluating docked ligands(17). We found that a mesh constructed approximately two van der Waals radii from binding site atoms was ideal for displaying steric effects. However, in order to display the chemical features of the binding site, additional algorithms were needed. A number of different properties of the protein surface were calculated using high resolution protein crystal structures. This large sample of experimental data was used to measure the correlation between the type of ligand atom and a calculated property of the nearest binding site surface. Properties such as the electrostatic potential and gradient were explored. However, the best correlation was obtained using a simple rule defining the hydrogen-bonding properties of the binding site. With this parameter, the surface could be divided into three separate zones representing the hydrophobic, hydrogen-bond acceptor and hydrogen-bond-donor properties of the binding site. Using the X-ray data of beta strands from the interior of proteins, the percentage of hydrophobic ligand atoms found to lie closest to the hydrophobic protein surface was 91%. The equivalent scores for ligand hydrogen-acceptor atoms and hydrogen-donor atoms found at the corresponding complementarity zones were 94% and 91% respectively.

For GrowMol, the accessible surface representation was extended to include the entire binding site cavity. This type of representation is useful for the rapid evaluation of the potential contribution of each new atom to the growing structure. The binding site is divided into a grid at 0.25 Å intervals. Each grid point is encoded with information about the nearest binding site atom. If the grid point is too close to a binding site atom, it is classified as forbidden. Grid points in contact with binding site atoms are classified as either hydrophobic, hydrogen-bond acceptor, or hydrogen-bond donor. Grid points further removed from binding site atoms are classified as neutral.

The cut-off distances for the various zones of the binding site grid map were determined using crystal structures of thermolysin inhibitor complexes. Each inhibitor was evaluated by determining how many of its carbon atoms occupy the binding site's hydrophobic zones, how many of its polar hydrogens are in the hydrogen bond acceptor zone, and how many of its hydrogen bond acceptors are in the hydrogen bond donating zone. A multiple linear regression was performed to correlate the log of the K_i of each inhibitor with the number of inhibitor/binding site hydrophobic contacts and hydrogen bonds. Cut-off distances for the various zones are described in the original paper. The r^2 for the regression was 0.94.

In the final evaluation (described below), the structures generated by GrowMol are energy minimized in the active site. Therefore, to test the effect of energy minimization, the nine thermolysin inhibitors were minimized in the binding site using QXP, a new docking program developed by one of us (Colin McMartin) (18) . Each structure was then evaluated in the grid box. The correlation between the log of Ki and the number of favorable contacts was now found to have an r^2 of 0.8. This decrease in correlation was not entirely unexpected as the parameterization of the accessible surface on which these rules were originally developed was based on high resolution X-ray structures.

We do not claim that this method can be used to reliably predict binding affinities. However, these results indicate a strong relationship between binding affinity and the number of favorable contacts between ligand and binding site atoms in this enzyme.

Molecular generation. The first step for generating molecules is the selection of a root atom by the user from which the new molecules will be grown. The root atom can be a single atom positioned in the target binding site or it can be an atom that is part of an already existing ligand to be optimized by GrowMol.

GrowMol then computes a series of "growth points" for this atom which are vectors representing energetically acceptable positions where new atoms can be positioned. For subsequent atoms, the "growth points" represent positions which will place the new atom in low energy conformations relative to previously grown segments. "Growth points" are computed using a lookup table based on the rotational isomeric states appropriate for that atom.

In step 2, GrowMol randomly selects one of the growth points for the position of the next atom. The type of atom to be placed at this growth point is also randomly selected from a small library of atoms and fragments consisting of C, N, -N=, O, O-, S, H, C=O, N-H, benzene and a five-membered aromatic ring with a nitrogen in one of the five positions. The selected atom or fragment is then constructed at the growth point using bond length and bond angles from the MM2 force field(19). The new atom(s) is evaluated and accepted or rejected depending on its degree of complementarity to the binding site, using Boltzmann statistics (for details see ref. 2). If the new atom is in the forbidden zone, it will be rejected and the growth point erased. If the new atom is in one of the allowed zones, a complementarity score is assigned and a Metropolis-like sampling criterion is used to decide if the new atom is to be retained and added to the growing chain. The probability of retaining a new atom is given by the Boltzmann factor:

$$BF=\exp(\text{-complementary score}/RT)$$

If the atom is accepted, it is connected to the growing chain and new growth points are computed. The program returns to step 2. If the atom is rejected the growth point is replaced and the program returns to step 2. This procedure biases the "growth" of atoms with a high degree of complementarity to the binding site but allows for the occasional inclusion of atoms which are not complementary but which may be necessary to allow for atoms with excellent complementarity to be generated further along the chain. The entire procedure continues until the user specified number of atoms and molecules has been grown.

Evaluation. GrowMol can rapidly generate large numbers of structures. (For example, it took 4 minutes 44 seconds to generate 1000 structures with 15 atoms in a binding site using a Silicon Graphics R10,000.) Once a set of structures has been generated, they can be evaluated and ranked for visualization. Two criteria are used: 1) favorable interactions with the binding site atoms (expressed as the number of favorable contacts) and 2) the internal molecular mechanics energy of the bound structures.

The evaluation begins with identification of the structures with a user specified minimal degree of complementarity, i.e. at least 3 hydrophobic contacts and at least 2 hydrogen bonds. These structures are then subjected to energy minimization in the active site and energy minimization in the absence of the binding site using the QXP docking program. (18) The difference between the energy of the bound conformation, and the energy of the conformation minimized outside of the binding site is taken as an initial measure of the ligand strain energy.

The ligand strain energy is used as a measure of how well the structure fits into the binding site cavity. Structures with high strain energies are discarded during the evaluation procedure.

After energy minimization, the structures are evaluated by a second grid box which has more stringent requirements for complementarity. Next the structures are clustered into families of structurally and chemically similar molecules. From each cluster, the structure with the highest degree of complementarity and the lowest strain energy is selected. This final set of structures is now ready for visual examination. This procedure was used to analyze a large set of potential inhibitors generated in the thermolysin binding site. 22,000 structures were generated. At the end of the evaluation procedure, the best 302 structures had been identified.

Applications. Enzymes are "designed" by nature to bind to the transition state of a substrate. We were intrigued by the question: how many other molecules, significantly different from the natural substrate, could also bind to a given enzyme? To explore this question, we used GrowMol to determine just how many structures complementary to the S1' and S2' subsites of thermolysin could be generated by this program. The binding site atoms were obtained from the structure of thermolysin bound with ZGPLL(20). This structure, labeled 5TMN, was obtained from the

Brookhaven Protein Data Bank(21). The S1' and S2' subsites are the best defined pockets of the thermolysin binding site and X-ray structures of small inhibitors which only use this part of the binding site are available. Known thermolysin inhibitors display a variety of different zinc binding groups. For this study, a sulfur atom which binds to the catalytic zinc ion was selected to be the root atom. The position of the sulfur, as well as that of the first growth point, were taken from the X-ray structure of thiorphan bound to thermolysin(22, 23). In this study, we decided to probe the site using aliphatic thiols, and, therefore, a carbon was selected for the first guest atom.

Three large sets of structures were generated: 50,000 with an average of 12.0 atoms each, 50,000 with an average of 13.8 atoms and 72,000 with 18.7 atoms. Table 1 summarizes the results.

Table 1

Number of Unique Structures found in Binding Site of Thermolysin

average no. of atoms	no. of structures	no. of unique structures	replication *rate*[a]	α^b
12.0	50 000	3938	12.7	1.99
13.8	50 000	10 543	4.7	1.96
18.7	72 000	39 680	1.8	1.76

[a]The number of structures divided by the number of unique structures found.

[b]Measure of diversity: number of unique structures=$\alpha^{(\text{number of atoms})}$.

As shown in table 1, the number of unique structures found increases with the number of atoms in each molecule as a result of a combinatorial explosion. The number of unique structures might be expected to increase as an exponential function of the number of atoms in the molecule:

$$N_{\text{unique}} = \alpha^{\text{Number of atoms}}$$

The value of α was found to be close to 2 (1.99 and 1.96) for the first two sets and somewhat lower for the third set (1.76). This lower value is very likely due to insufficient sampling of this set of relatively large structures. The parameter α is useful to predict the number of unique structures which GrowMol could generate for a given size of molecule. For example, for a molecule with 30 heavy atoms, GrowMol is expected to generate approximately one billion unique structures.

To evaluate the structure generating and scoring algorithms used by GrowMol, the reported thiol inhibitors of thermolysin were compared to structures generated by GrowMol. A literature search conducted at the time of this study (1994) revealed fourteen thiol thermolysin inhibitors. Six of these compounds are alpha thiols. At that time no experimental data was available revealing the binding modes of alpha thiol inhibitors of zinc metallo-proteases. The (S) isomer of retro-thiorphan is a weakly-binding inhibitor with a K_i of 94 μM and was, therefore, also excluded. Figure 1 shows a comparison between the known inhibitors and the similar structures generated by GrowMol.

Most significantly, GrowMol spontaneously generated both the (S) and (R) isomer of thiorphan(23), the 10-membered macrocyclic lactam(24) and a ten membered benzo-fused macrocycle similar to the very potent eleven membered benzo-fused macrocycle(25). Retro- thiorphan(23) could not be generated using the fixed sulfur from thiorphan. However, when a ensemble of root atoms were generated using dynamics, GrowMol was also successful at "growing" this inhibitor.

GrowMol also generated a large number of structures different from known inhibitors. Reference 2 and 3 show examples of some of these novel structures.

Although the generation of structures equal or closely similar to known inhibitors is a good way to evaluate a de novo computer program, the true test of such a program is the synthesis and experimental verification that the novel molecule indeed binds to the target receptor as predicted. Unfortunately none of the novel inhibitors generated in the binding site of thermolysin have to our knowledge been synthesized.

Application to pepsin. In collaboration with Prof. Daniel Rich at the University of Wisconsin, Madison, GrowMol was used to discover novel molecular scaffolds for designing peptide-mimetic inhibitors of aspartic proteases. The X-ray structure of A66702 complexed to pepsin(26) was used as a starting point (figure 2). First, GrowMol was tested to see if the program could generate structures similar to known inhibitors. The progam generated a series of known cyclic inhibitors in which the side chains in the P1 and P3 inhibitors subsites are connected(27).

Next GrowMol was used to generate novel structures using the hydroxyl oxygen of statine as the root atom. 50,000 - 100,000 structures were rapidly generated. These were evaluated, clustered and ranked, resulting in 200 - 400 distinct strutures that were examined for synthetic feasibility by the chemists. One of the interesting structures GrowMol generated is shown in the figure 3 below. Structure 1 was simplified, resulting in a series of compounds for synthesis to test this GrowMol prediction. The first compound to be synthesized was Structure 2, the cyclohexanol derivative. This compound did not inhibit pepsin at the the highest concentration tested (400 μM). When docked into the pepsin binding site with the QXP program (figure 4), two important interactions, present in A66702, were found to be absent in **2**: a hydrophobic group in the S2 pepsin subsite and a hydrogen bond to the loop which covers the binding site. According to our docking experiments, the addition of a phenyl to occupy the position of the pyrole of structure 1, would occupy the S2 subsite. Addition of this moiety resulted in compound **3** which did inhibit pepsin, with a K_i of 4.9. The

Known Inhibitors	Experimental Potency K_i, μM	Estimated Potency K_i, μM	GROWMOL Structures	Estimated Potency K_i, μM	Estimated Potency K_i, μM Before Energy Minimization In Active Site
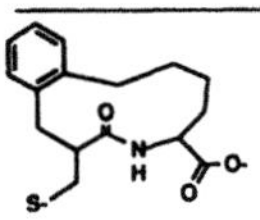	0.019[a]	0.043	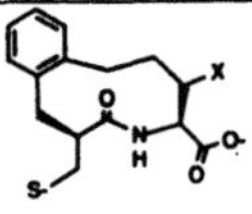	0.30	0.78
			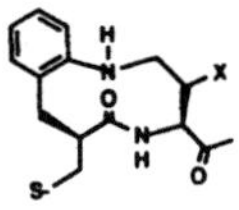	0.30	2.0
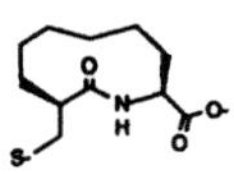	3.8[b]	5.4	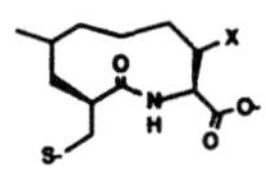	0.30	2.0
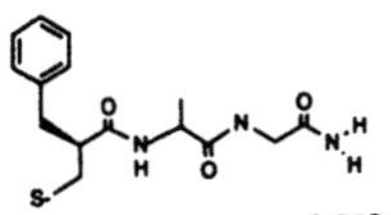	0.75[c]	0.78	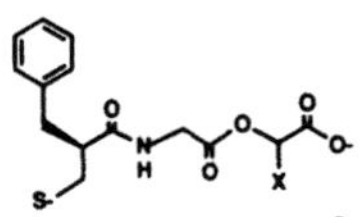	0.12	0.89
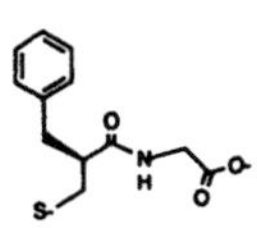	1.8[d]	0.11	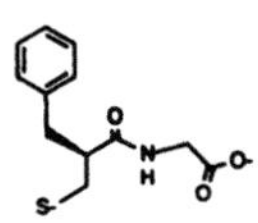	0.11	5.3
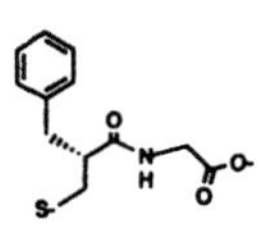	3.0[d]	0.77	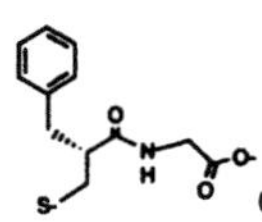	0.77	97.8
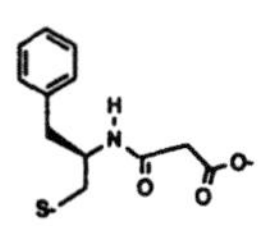	2.3[d]	0.77	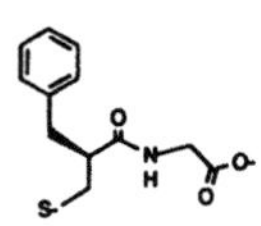	0.11	5.3
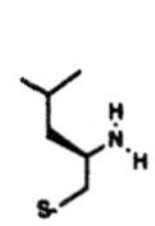	5.3[e]	85	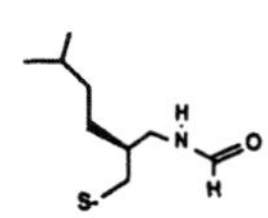	12.3	32.4
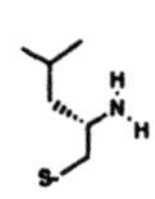	52[f]	224	none		

FIG. 1. [a]*See ref 25.* [b]*See ref 24.* [c]*See ref 27.* [d]*See ref 22.* [e]*This compound binds to thermolysin in a noncompetitive manner, and, therefore, cannot be compared with the rest of the potency data.(28).* *f See ref 28. Comparison between thiol inhibitors of known potency and structures generated by GrowMol. Potency estimates based on complementarity to the binding site are shown for the known inhibitors as well as the GrowMol structures. To show the effect of optimization by energy minimization in the active site, the potency estimates* before *energy minimization are also given.*

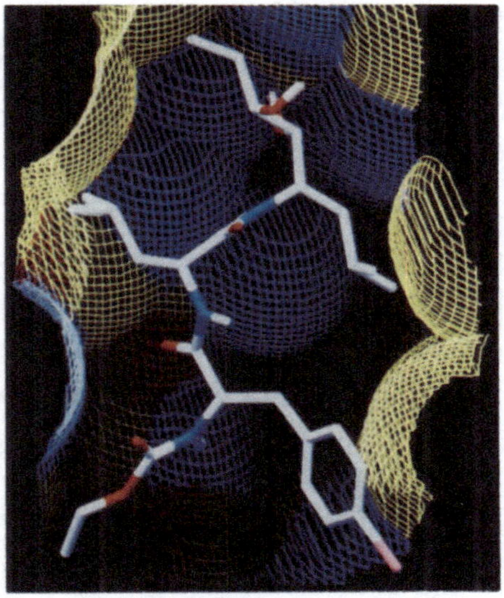

FIG. 2. *The active site of porcine pepsin with A66702, from the crystal structure of the A66702/pepsin complex. The binding site atoms are covered with the Lee and Richards accessible surface. The yellow mesh indicates hydrophobic areas of the binding site. Blue mesh covers hydrogen bond acceptors and red mesh covers hydrogen bond donors.*

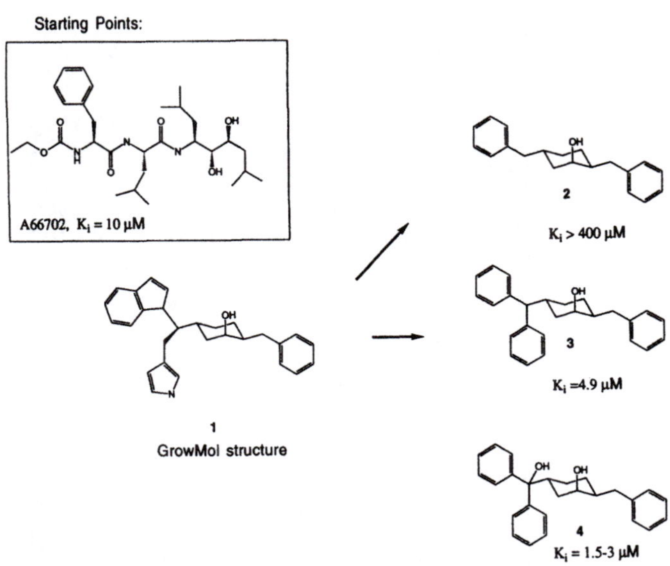

FIG. 3. *The crystal structure of pepsin complexed with A66702 was used to generate novel structures to complement the pepsin binding site. One of the hydroxyl groups (that on the left) of A66702 was used as the root atom. Structure* **1** *was one of the structures generated by GrowMol that was simplified for synthesis. Compounds* **2**, **3**, *and* **4** *were synthesized. The experimentally determined* K_i*'s are given.*

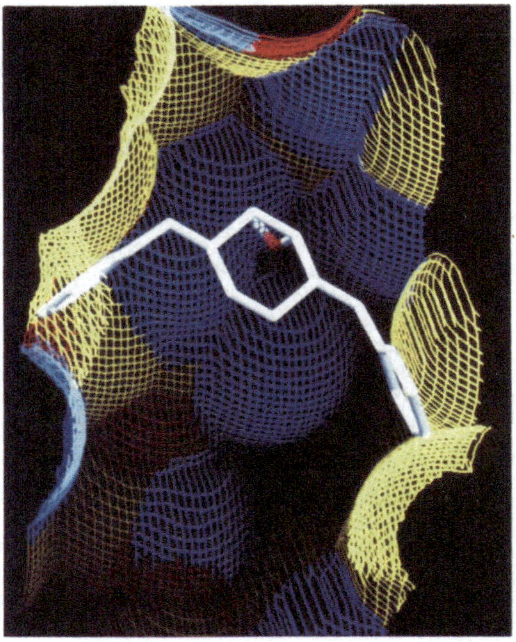

FIG. 4. *Compound **2** docked into the porcine pepsin binding site.*

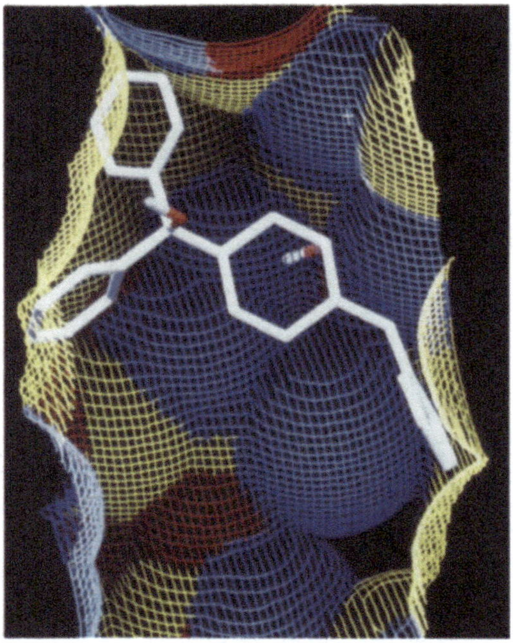

FIG. 5. *Compound **4** docked into the porcine pepsin binding site.*

second hydroxyl group of **4** is predicted by docking experiments to form a hydrogen bond with the loop which covers part of the pepsin binding site (figure 5). Compound **4** was synthesized and found to have a K_i=1.5 to 3 μM. This compound is of special interest because it contains no nitrogen, and at the time the Rich group began this work, no tight-binding inhibitors of pepsin devoid of nitrogen were known.

Conclusions

GrowMol has now been used in a variety of different binding sites including thermolysin, stromelysin, collagenase, pepsin, HIV protease, thrombin, cathepsin B, purine nucleoside phosphorylase (PNP) and cyclin-dependent protein kinase 2 (CDK2) In each of these cases the program generated structures similar to, as well as different from, known inhibitors.

It has been demonstrated in thermolysin that GrowMol is useful for identifying large numbers of highly diverse molecules that are structurally, chemically and energetically complementary to an enzyme binding site. Such libraries are useful to medicinal chemists who can extract suitable potential lead structures for further design and synthesis.

It has now been shown by Rich et al. that some of these compounds which show no similarity at all to the natural peptidic substrate, inhibit the target enzyme, pepsin. This is one of the first examples of the successful use of a *de novo* computer program leading to an active, entirely novel enzyme inhibitor.

Acknowledgment. The development of GrowMol and the study on thermolysin were conducted at Ciba-Geigy (now Novartis). The authors wish to thank Drs. Wayne Guida and Frank Clarke for their support and encouragement.

REFERENCES

1. E. Fischer, *Ber. Dtsch. Ges.* **27**, 2985 (1894).
2. R. S. Bohacek, C. McMarin, *J. Amer. Chem .Soc.* **116**, 5560–5571 (1994).
3. R. Bohacek, C. McMartin, *Nature Medicine* **1**, 177–178 (1995).
4. D. H. Rich, R. S. Bohacek, N. A. Dales, P. Glunz, A. S. Ripka, *Chimia* **51**, 45–47 (1997).
5. Y. Nishibata, A. Itai, *Tetrahedron*, **47**, 8985–8990 (1991).
6. J. B. Moon, W. J. Howe, *Proteins: Struct., Funct., Genet.* **11**, 314–328 (1991).
7. H.-J. Boehm, *Current Opin. in Biotechnology* **7**, 433–436 (1996).
8. H.-J. Boehm, *J. Comput. Aided Mol. Des.* **6**, 61–78 (1992).
9. A. Miranker, M. Karplus, *Proteins* **11**, 29–34 (1991).
10. A. Miranker, M. Karplus, *Proteins* **23**, 472–490 (1995).
11. D. A. Pearlman, M. A. Murcko, *J. Med. Chem.* **10**, 1184–1193 (1993).
12. D. A. Pearlman, M. A. Murcko, *J. Med. Chem.* **39**, 1651–1663 (1996).
13. A. Calfisch, A. Miranker, M. Karplus, *J. Med. Chem.* **36**, 2142–2167 (1993).
14. A. Calfisch, *J. Comput. Aided Mol. Des.* **10**, 372–396 (1996).
15. D. K. Gehlhaar, et al., *J. Med. Chem.*, **38**, 466–472 (1995).
16. S. H. Rotstein, M. A. Murcko, *J. Med. Chem.* **36** 1700–1710 (1993).
17. R. S. Bohacek, C. McMartin, *J. Med. Chem.* **35**, 1671–1684 (1992).

18. C. McMartin, R. Bohacek, *J. Comput-Aided Mol. Des.* **9**, 237–250 (1997).
19. N. L. Allinger, *J. Am. Chem. Soc.* **99**, 8127–8140 (1977).
20. P. A. Bartlett, C. K. Marlowe, *Science* **235**, 569–571 (1987).
21. F. C. Berstein, et al., *J. Mol. Biol.* **112**, 535–542 (1977).
22. S. L. Roderick, M. C. Fournie-Zaluski, B. P. Roques, B. W. Matthews, *Biochemistry* **28**, 1493–1497 (1989).
23. T. Benchetrit, M. C. Fournie-Zaluski, B. P. Roques, *Biophys. Res. Commun.* **147**, 1034–1040 (1987).
24. L. J. MacPherson, et al., *J. Med. Chem.* **36**, 3821–3828 (1993).
25. G. M. Ksander, et al., *J. Med. Chem.* **40**, 495–505 (1997).
26. L. Chen, et al., *Acta Crystallogr., Sect. B* **48**, 476 (1992).
27. D. J. Rich, R. S. Bohacek, N. A. Dales, P. Glunz, A. S. Ripka, *Combinatorial design and combinatorial synthesis of enzyme inhibitors*, Actualites de Chimie Therapeutic-22e serie (Elseveir, Amsterdam, 1996).
28. D. S. Pickering, M. V. Kirshna, D. C. Miller, W. W. Chan, *Arch. Biochem. Biophys.* **239**, 368–374 (1985).

DEDUCING OBJECTIVE SITE MODELS BY MIXED INTEGER PROGRAMMING

GORDON M. CRIPPEN*

Abstract. One of the most challenging problems in computer-aided drug design is deducing one or more models of a binding site solely from the known chemical structures and measured binding affinities of a few small molecules. In particular, the X-ray crystal structure of the receptor is not known. The main difficulty is deciding how the different ligands are supposed to bind to the common site, especially when they differ substantially in chemical structure. The usual approach is to first guess or use some separate algorithm to superimpose at least the active compounds on one another and then adjust other parameters associated with the model to fit the observed affinities without further altering the proposed alignment. We have explored a long series of algorithms that instead consider the many ways each ligand could fit in the site, and then adjust the site parameters until the best way each molecule can fit has a calculated binding affinity that agrees with experiment. Thus each of the different binding modes of each molecule is some sort of constraint on the geometry and energetic features of the site model. Here we show how to unite the geometric and energetic constraints of the many different binding modes of conformationally flexible ligands in a common framework of mixed integer programming. When applied to the standard test case of corticosteroid binding globulin, even a single compound as the training set can produce a variety of site models having considerable predictive power.

1. Introduction. Most ordinary drugs consist of small, synthetic, organic molecules that bring about their desired biological effect by specific binding to some cleft or cavity in a macromolecule, typically a protein. For example, the drug may be an inhibitor of some particular enzyme in the body that works by filling up the active site so that the enzyme can't catalyze some reaction associated with the disease state. While the delivery of the drug to the vicinity of the target binding site can be engineered somewhat, the last $10^5 \AA$ of the journey depend on random diffusion through the solvent. In most cases, an equilibrium is established between drug molecules (or "ligands") sampling all sorts of positions, orientations, and internal molecular conformations in the isotropic solvent and ligands in all sorts of orientations and conformations in the very different environment set up by the binding site. Often there is one position, relative orientation, and conformation of the ligand within the binding site (the ligand's binding "mode") that is so much more favorable in free energy over alternative modes that almost all bound ligand molecules adopt it. In this case, an X-ray crystal structure of the protein complexed with the ligand would clearly show exactly how it fits into the cleft. Meanwhile the receptor protein usually makes only small accommodations to fit different ligands, giving rise to sometimes great differences in binding strength brought about by small changes in the chemical structures of the ligands. The causes of the strength of binding for the optimal mode can usually be broken down into

*College of Pharmacy, University of Michigan, Ann Arbor, Michigan 48109-1065.

specific hydrogen bonds between ligand and site, electrostatic interactions between the ligand and the inhomogeneous field set up by the protein, and general desolvation of at least portions of the ligand where it fits tightly against the hard walls of the site.

Experimentally measuring the binding affinity of a few compounds competing for the same site on a protein is much easier than determining the three-dimensional structure of that protein, so usually all we have to go on are the chemical structures of the ligands, their observed binding affinities, and some reasonable exploration of the allowed range of conformations by standard molecular mechanics methods. Without building in a lot of assumptions about how each ligand can best fit into the site, can we deduce at least a low-resolution model of the shape of the binding cavity and the different energetic environments that ligand atoms experience in different part of it? Here we describe the computational methods behind EGSITE2, the latest in a long series of programs that tackle this problem. [1,2] Even if we assume the observed binding strength of a particular mode can be approximated by some linear function of adjustable energy parameters associated with the site model, the geometry of the site is usually thought of in nonlinear terms, and then there is the combinatorial feature of having many different binding modes possible for each ligand. EGSITE2 exploits techniques from linear programming to convert all this into a series of mixed integer programs (MIP) that are feasible to solve.

2. Methods.

2.1. Input data. Molecule i has experimental binding affinity in the interval $[L_i, U_i]$, preferably expressed on a scale proportional to $-\Delta G_{\text{bind}}$, the free energy of transfer from the site into the solvent. Thus zero corresponds to being in bulk solvent, and large, positive values correspond to tighter, more favorable binding to the site. For estimating the binding affinity of any given mode, we assign to each atom, independent of conformation, three physiochemical parameters (p_{hp}, p_{MR}, p_{ch}): an atomic contribution to $\log P$ and to the molar refractivity, [6] and a Gasteiger partial charge. [7] The relatively low-energy conformations of each isolated ligand are explored by standard software, such as MM2 within MSI's Cerius^2 software [4]. The result was summarized in terms of several alternative conformations, depending on how flexible the ligand was.

2.2. Site definition. Since the real ligand chooses between the solvent environment and the various environments offered in different parts of the real binding site, let the site model consist of a small number of discrete regions, the first one always representing the solvent, and the others corresponding to different pockets in the receptor. For each region there are three adjustable interaction parameters (S_{hp}, S_{MR}, S_{ch}), corresponding to the fixed hydrophobicity, polarity, and charge properties of the atoms. We fix $\vec{S} = 0$ for the solvent region. To simplify notation, concatenate all the region interaction parameters into a list of variables S_k, so that if for a particular binding mode the sum of the corresponding fixed atomic physiochemical property values for those atoms in that region is p_k, then the calculated binding affinity is $\sum_k S_k p_k$. The geometry of the site is expressed as G_{Ukl} = the upper bound on the distance between a point in region k and a point in region l, and G_{Lkl} = the corresponding lower bound, taken over all pairs of the n_r regions. We fix all $G_{Ukl} = \infty$ for $k =$ the solvent region. Trivially, $G_{Lkk} = 0$ for all k. The regions are viewed as non-overlapping, but not necessarily covering all space. For technical reasons, we rescale all distances that may occur in the problem so that interregion distances are always even integers, and distances between subsets of atoms are odd integers.

2.3. Binding modes. A binding *mode* of a ligand molecule to a site model constitutes a discrete choice of one of the allowed conformations, and which atoms are assigned to lie in which regions. This amounts to assigning atoms to mutually exclusive subsets, so for that chosen conformation, d_{Ukl} = the upper bound on the distance between an atom that is supposed to lie in region k and an atom that lies in region l, and d_{LKl} is the corresponding lower bound on interatomic distances. Any molecule always has available the trivial binding mode where all atoms in any conformation are in one subset assigned to the solvent region. A mode is denoted as *disallowed* with respect to a given site if any $d_{Ukl} > G_{Ukl}$ or $d_{Lkl} < G_{Lkl}$. With respect to energetics, the ith ligand's mode is *suboptimal* if $\sum_k S_k p_k < L_i$, *superoptimal* if $\sum_k S_k p_k > U_i$, and *in-range* if $\sum_k S_k p_k \in [L_i, U_i]$.

2.4. Basis set of modes. Suppose we have a set of several modes for each ligand we are considering. In order to express relationships between the various constraints by which the basis determines the site, we will need standard Boolean variables having values of either 1 for true or 0 for false. For the ith mode in the basis, let Y_i = the Boolean variable for being in-range, g_i = Boolean allowed geometrically, and h_{ij} = Boolean disallowed for the jth reason out of n_{ih} possible reasons. Clearly n_{ih} depends on the number of subsets in mode i, which in turn is no greater than n_r. Let M be a large positive number that is bigger than any experimental binding affinity or the diameter of any molecule in any conformation. Then the following Boolean expressions must be satisfied:

$$(d_{Ukl} + 1)g_i - G_{Ukl} \leq 0 \tag{2.1}$$

i.e., an allowed mode must not violate upper bounds on any variable interregion distances kl, but if the mode is disallowed, these constraints have no effect;

$$d_{Lkl} + (M - d_{Lkl} + 1)g_i \leq M \tag{2.2}$$

i.e., similarly, an allowed mode must not violate lower bounds on any variable interregion distances kl, but if the mode is disallowed, these constraints also have no effect;

$$(-d_{Ukl} + 1 + M)h_{ij} + G_{Ukl} \leq M \tag{2.3}$$

i.e., a disallowed mode may violate some upper bound on interregion distances, but if the mode is not disallowed for this reason, the constraint has no effect;

$$(d_{Lkl} + 1)h_{ij} - G_{Lkl} \leq 0 \tag{2.4}$$

i.e., another reason a mode may be disallowed is for violating some lower bound on interregion distances, but if it is not disallowed on this account, the constraint has no effect;

$$-\sum_k p_k S_k + (L_i + M)Y_i \leq M \tag{2.5}$$

i.e., any in-range mode must have calculated binding affinity at least as strong as the weakest observed value, but if it is not in-range, the calculated affinity has no lower limit;

$$\sum_k p_k S_k + (M - L_i)g_i + (L_i - U_i)Y_i \leq M \tag{2.6}$$

i.e., no allowed mode can be superoptimal, but an allowed mode that is not in-range must bind more weakly than the observed lower limit;

$$\sum h_{ij} + n_{hi} g_i \leq n_{hi} \tag{2.7}$$

i.e., if a mode is allowed, it cannot be disallowed for any reason;

$$-\sum h_{ij} - g_i \leq -1 \tag{2.8}$$

i.e., either a mode is allowed or it is disallowed for at least one reason;

$$Y_i \leq g_i \tag{2.9}$$

i.e., an in-range mode must be geometrically allowed;

$$-\sum_{\substack{\text{modes of} \\ \text{molecule}}} Y_i \leq -1 \tag{2.10}$$

i.e., at least one mode for each molecule must be in-range.

2.5. Algorithm. (1) Given n_r chosen by the user and a training set of ligands, the algorithms starts by building a basis consisting of typically ten modes for each molecule, discovered in a random search that selects those ten that are maximally different from one another in terms of the aggregate physiochemical properties p_k of the subsets, and the subset geometry, d_{Ukl} and d_{Lkl} for all kl. The partitioning of the atoms in these initial modes is done assuming the least geometrically restrictive site geometry, namely $G_{Ukl} = M$ and $G_{Lkl} = 0$ for all kl.

(2) For only the initial basis set of modes, solve the mixed integer program (MIP) corresponding to eqs. 2.1–2.10 for all modes. For the corresponding linear program (LP), the default variable bounds are $0 \leq Y$, g, $h \leq 1$ for all the Boolean variables, $-M \leq S_k \leq M$ for all the $3(n_r - 1)$ interaction parameters, and $0 \leq G_{ULkl} \leq M$ for all the adjustable geometric parameters. The objective of the LP is to minimize $\sum_{k,l}(G_{Lkl} - G_{Ukl})$, which biases the solutions toward unrestrictive geometry, i.e. large diameter regions that touch one another. We solve the LP using the standard commercial software, Cplex. [8] Then solving the MIP consists of a standard depth-first branch and bound search over all combinations of choices of the Boolean variable values 0 and 1, eliminating a branch when the associated LP is infeasible. It turns out that some of the Boolean variables are much more influential in determining the values of others. The binary search tree is therefore carefully ordered in advance to consider these variables first. The search stops at the first feasible MIP solution, or it declares the MIP infeasible when 10^4 nodes have been visited, or the whole search tree has been eliminated, whichever comes first. Of course there is always the risk that no solution will be found to the MIP simply because the right combination of modes was not available in the basis, but even with the initial basis of only 10 modes per ligand, this has not been a problem.

(3) The candidate site is repeatedly challenged by searching for superoptimal modes of any training set ligand to add to the basis. If any can be found, a restricted MIP holding the site geometry constant is solved (eqs. 2.5, 2.6, and 2.10). This involves only the allowed modes. The objective of the associated LP is the maximization of the sum of the calculated binding affinities of all modes. As the basis grows, the time required to solve the MIP increases, but in practice, the majority of the time goes into the searching for superoptimal modes. Eventually either the MIP becomes infeasible, or no superoptimal mode of any training ligand can be found. In the latter case, the site geometry and final energetic parameters constitute a solution. In either case, this choice of site geometry, $G_{ULkl,old}$, is eliminated from further consideration by adding the cutting plane

$$\sum G_{Ukl} - \sum G_{Lkl} \leq \sum G_{Ukl,old} - \sum G_{Lkl,old} - 1 \tag{2.11}$$

to the full MIP in step 2. Given that the objective of that LP is to maximize the left hand side of this inequality, such cutting planes probably do not eliminate other solutions. Eventually, the full MIP becomes infeasible due to all the cutting planes, and the search terminates. If no solutions were found, the user can increment n_r by 1 and try again. It is generally a good policy to start with $n_r = 2$ and work up.

(4) In step 3 and in making predictions, the essential part is searching for the best, perhaps superoptimal, mode of a given molecule in a given site. For all the different conformations summarizing the flexibility of the molecule, systematically try subdividing the atoms into $1, ..., n_r$ subsets. For a given choice of conformation and number of subsets, systematically try all distinct assignments of subsets of site regions. For each assignment, try 10 randomly chosen combinations of atoms to serve as subset "centers", which will determine which atoms belong to which subsets and therefore the calculated binding affinity. Any change of one atom center at a time that improves the binding is accepted until no further improvement can be made (i.e., a simple greedy algorithm that depends on the starting choice of centers and therefore requires multiple random starts). The partitioning of all the atoms into disjoint subsets given a particular choice of center atoms goes as follows. Initially put each atom into the subset corresponding to the closest center, provided the distance from atom to center is less than $G_{Ukk}/2$, where the subset has been assigned to region k. This may leave some atoms assigned to no subset because the choice of center atom was geometrically far from the centroid of the final subset of atoms. Order the unassigned atoms according to increasing minimal distance to assigned atoms. Then attempt to add the first unassigned atom to the subset, if any, that is closest to it such that the resulting subset diameter $d_{Ukk} < G_{Ukk}$ of the corresponding site region. Then go to the second unassigned atom in the ordered list, etc. Of course, the diameter of a subset of atoms is taken to be the maximal distance between any two of the member atoms. In the end, some atoms may remain unassigned, implying that this mode is incompatible with the given site geometry, so the mode is flagged with a large, negative calculated binding affinity to ensure that the trivial mode of being completely out in the solvent scores better.

2.6. Site assessment and predictions. Clearly, the computational requirements increase rapidly as the number of ligands in the training set increases, especially if the molecules are large and conformationally flexible. On the other hand, deducing a site on the basis of a small training set generally leads to numerous solutions producing a wide variety of predictions. If we designate a passive set of ligands beyond the training set, they can be used to test solutions, and those giving large predictive errors on the passive set can be discarded. Here the error is taken to be the sum over the passive set of the absolute values of any over/under-predictions.

Finally, all the accepted solutions are used to predict the optimal binding mode and its affinity for every ligand in a test set. If there is more than one solution, each ligand has an interval of predictions on the

TABLE 1
Observed and Calculated Binding of CBG and TBG with Steroids 1–31.

cmpd.[a]	CBG obsd.[b]	CBG calcd.
1	[5.28,7.28]	[c][7.28,7.80]xs
2	[4.00,6.00]	[d][5.85,6.11]xs
3	[4.00,6,00]	[d][6.11,6.26]hi
4	[4.76,6.76]	[d][5.44,6.87]xs
5	[4.61,6.61]	[d][5.56,5.94]ok
6	[6.88,8.88]	[d][7.15,7.23]ok
7	[6.88,8.88]	[d][7.54,7.63]ok
8	[5.89,7.89]	[d][7.34,7.37]ok
9	[4.00,6.00]	[6.25,6.51]hi
10	[6.65,8.65]	[6.78,6.85]ok
11	[6.88,8.88]	[6.99,7.15]ok
12	[4.92,6.92]	[5.56,5.94]ok
13	[4.00,6.00]	[5.26,5.64]ok
14	[4.00,6.00]	[5.94,6.02]xs
15	[4.00,6.00]	[4.97,5.47]ok
16	[4.22,6.22]	[5.56,6.41]xs
17	[4.22,6.22]	[6.62,6.75]hi
18	[4.00,6.00]	[6.82,7.01]hi
19	[6.38,8.38]	[6.38,6.55]ok
20	[6.74,8.74]	[6.45,6.81]xs
21	[5.72,7.72]	[5.73,6.06]ok
22	[6.51,8.51]	[7.70,7.84]ok
23	[6.55,8.55]	[8.24,9.27]xs
24	[5.78,7.78]	[6.31,6.71]ok
25	[6.20,8.20]	[7.15,7.23]ok
26	[5.11,7.11]	[5.47,5.76]ok
27	[5.25,7.25]	[6.99,7.44]xs
28	[6.12,8.12]	[6.20,6.78]ok
29	[5.82,7.82]	[5.84,6.20]ok
30	[6.69,8.69]	[7.82,7.85]ok
31	[4.80,6.80]	[7.79,8.07]hi

[a] Fig. 1.[b] $\log K_{\text{diss}} \pm 1.0$, ref. 9. [c]active training set. [d]passive training set.

affinity scale, $[L_{i,\text{pred}}, U_{i,\text{pred}}]$, namely the minimal and maximal prediction over all solutions. The composite prediction is correct if $L_{i,\text{pred}} \geq L_i$ and $U_{i,\text{pred}} \leq U_i$, low if $U_{i,\text{pred}} < L_i$, high if $L_{i,\text{pred}} > U_i$, and otherwise "excess" if the predicted interval overlaps the experimental interval but

TABLE 2
The four CBG 2-Region Site Models.

Model	Region Geometry ($\AA$)[a]		Region Energetics HP	MR	charge
solvent	∞	∞	0.00	0.00	0.00
1	0	∞	−0.42	0.09	0.50
2	0	∞	−0.22	0.08	1.27
3	0	∞	−0.26	0.08	0.67
4	0	13.7	−0.27	0.08	1.68

[a] Each of the four models consists of a solvent region described in the first row of the table and one binding pocket described by one of the other four subsequent rows. Thus the geometry of the first model is given in terms of the 2×2 matrix of inter-region distances given in the first two rows.

extends beyond it, above and/or below.

3. Results.

3.1. Binding to CBG. Here we tested EGSITE2 on the same set of 31 steroids binding to human corticosteroid binding globulin (CBG) [9] that has served as a benchmark for several computational methods. [1,11,12,13,14] The structures and numbering of the compounds is as in Jain et al., [14] and the set of conformers for each was derived as before, [1] except between six and nine of the lowest energy conformers were kept for each compound to represent conformational flexibility. Using only **1** as the active training set, along with **2–8** as passive training compounds, the program easily found its given limit of ten site models, each having only two regions. These represented a total of five different geometries, but those where the non-solvent region was not very large gave prediction errors on the passive set in the range of 0.89–2.95. The four best sites (Table 2) had errors of only 0.29–0.44. These were tested against the remaining 23 test compounds (Table 1), and also the active and passive compounds were checked for predicted binding, realizing that a renewed search for optimal binding modes may fail to find ones as good as those located in the training procedure, or it may discover superoptimal modes.

The one training compound, **1**, was overpredicted by 0.52 by one of the four models, but correctly predicted by the rest. Of the seven passive training compounds, four were correctly predicted, two has excess ranges, and one was high by 0.1. Of the 23 test compounds, 14 were correct, one was excess by 0.02, four were substantially in excess, and four were high. These results are summarized graphically in Fig. 2.

4. Conclusions. At first glance it may seem outrageous that on the basis of a single training compound, only four out of thirty were clearly mispredicted, and for six the predictions were neither clearly right nor wrong. Remember, however, that the training procedure ensures that there is at least one in-range mode and no superoptimal modes out of the enormous number possible for that one training compound. In other words, one compound may constitute many more than one constraint on the site model.

Experience with EGSITE2 continues to grow. Conceptually, the main advantage is to be able to treat both the continuous energetic and geometric features of the site model in a uniform way, while linking together the discrete set of different binding modes of the training molecules into one MIP. Very little user input is required, beyond the adjustable parameters governing how thorough various subproblems are searched. This is likely to be most effective in cases such as CBG, where a very low resolution model based on nonspecific interactions between ligand and site is sufficient. On the other hand, it would likely be very time-consuming for a data set that must be explained by several tightly localized hydrogen bonding interactions between the site and large, flexible molecules.

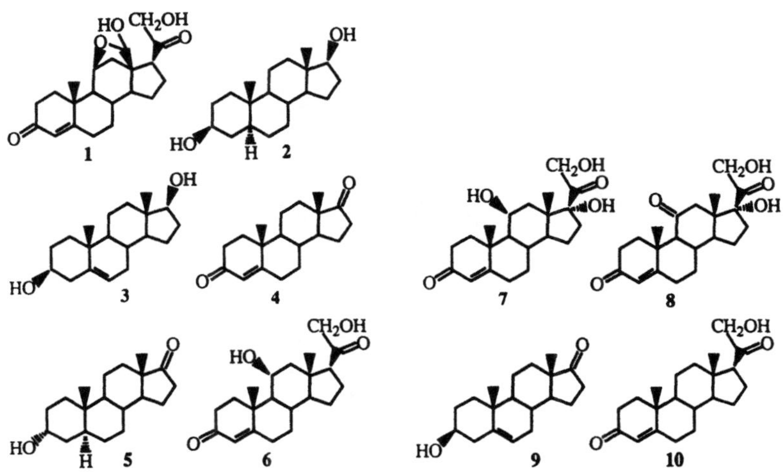

FIG. 1. *Steroid structures.*

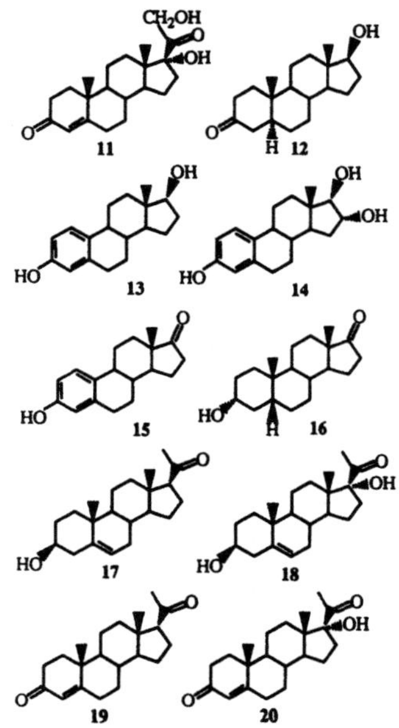

Fig. 1. (continued)

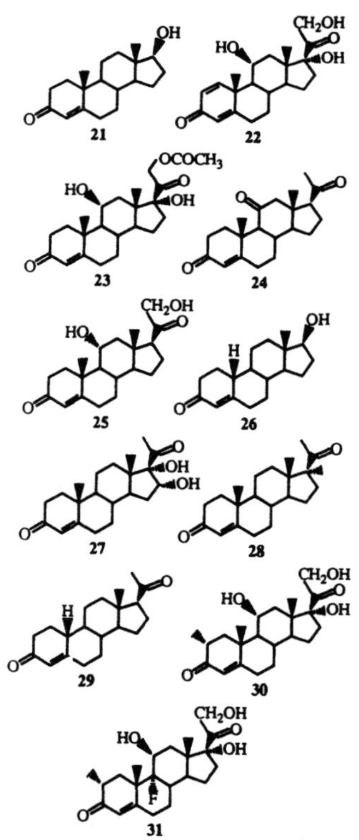

Fig.1. (continued)

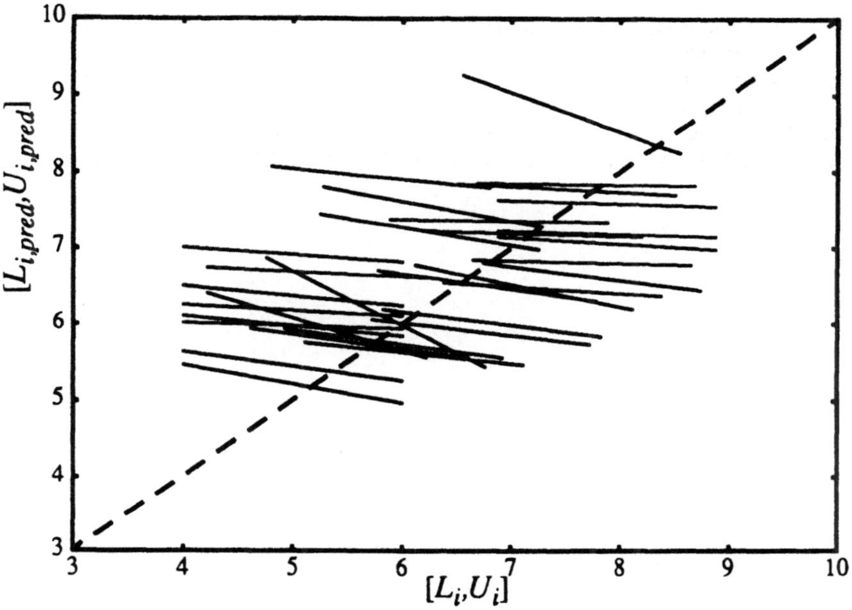

FIG. 2. *Observed vs. calculated binding of the 31 CBG ligands to four site models (Tables 1 and 2). Since both observed and calculated affinities are intervals, each compound is represented by a diagonal line segment running from* $(L_i, U_{i,pred})$ *to* $(U_i, L_{i,pred})$. *Any that cross the dashed line representing observed = calculated are correct predictions.*

REFERENCES

[1] SCHNITKER, J., GOLPALASWAMY, R., AND CRIPPEN, G.M., Objective models for steroid binding sites of human globulins, *J. Comp.-Aided Mol. Design*, 1997, 11, 93–110.

[2] CRIPPEN, G.M., Intervals and the deduction of drug binding site models, *J. Comp. Chem.*, 1995, 16, 486–500.

[3] BRADLEY, M., RICHARDSON, W., AND CRIPPEN, G.M., Deducing molecular similarity using Voronoi binding sites, *J. Chem. Inf. Comp. Sci.*, 1993, 33, 750–755.

[4] Molecular Simulations, Inc., 9685 Scranton Rd., San Diego, CA; http://www.msi.com.

[5] MAYO, S.L., OLAFSON, B.D., AND GODDARD, W.A., DREIDING: A generic force field for molecular simulations, *J. Phys. Chem.*, 1990, 94, 8897–8909.

[6] GHOSE, A.K., PRITCHETT, A., AND CRIPPEN, G.M., Atomic physico-chemical parameters for three dimensional structure directed quantitative structure-activity relationships III: Modeling hydrophobic interactions, *J. Comp. Chem.*, 1988, 9, 80–90.

[7] MORTIER, W.J., VAN GENECHTEN, K., AND GASTEIGER, J., *J. Amer. Chem. Soc.*, 1985, 107, 829.

[8] CPLEX Optimization, Inc., Suite 279, 930 Tahoe Blvd., Incline Village, NV; http://www.cplex.com.

[9] MICHELSON, K.E., FORSTHOEFEL, J., AND WESTPHAL, U., *Biochemistry*, 1981, 20, 6211–6218.

[10] DUNN, J.F., NISSULA, B.C., AND RODBARD, D., *J. Clin. Endocrin. Metab.*, 1981, 53, 58–68.

[11] Cramer, R.D., Patterson, D.E., and Bunce, J.D., *J. Am. Chem. Soc.*, 1988, 110, 5959.
[12] Kellogg, G.E., Semus, S.F., and Abraham, D.J., *J. Comp.-Aided Mol. Design*, 1991, 5, 545.
[13] Good, A.C., So, S.-S., and Richards, W.G., *J. Med. Chem.*, 1993, 36, 433.
[14] Jain, A.N., Koile, K., and Chapman, D., *J. Med. Chem.*, 1994, 37, 2315.

MOLECULAR DYNAMICS INFORMATION EXTRACTION

DENNIS SPROUS*, WEIDONG WANG*, GANESAN RAVISHANKER*
MATTHEW A. YOUNG*, AND DAVID L. BEVERIDGE*

Key words. MD, MD ToolChest 2.0, CURVES, phased A-tract DNA structure, Hagerman sequences

Abstract. MD-trajectories currently span nanoseconds of simulated time. The parameters most commonly presented in MD papers are RMS, energy and temperature presented as functions of time. These are easily obtained from a variety of sources, most commonly the output files of the simulation itself. However, the most critical structural parameters are not available directly from program output files, but require post processing. Typically, these parameters are specific for a given molecule type. Pucker angle and other helicoidals are important for DNA. Ramachandran plots are obviously relevant for proteins. Hydrogen bond distances would be relevant for a ligand-DNA or ligand-protein simulation. The various modeling packages normally incorporate an analysis program such as the *AMBER CARNAL* program. The *MD-ToolChest (MDTC)* suite of programs was designed to analyze data from a broad range of sources and can read trajectory files from *AMBER*, *GROMOS* and *CHARMm*. For DNA, its flagship program *dials_and_windows_dna* serves as a front end for passing coordinates to the*CURVES* (Lavery and Sklenar, 1996) program. Complete helicoidal parameters are presented as time series. For proteins, a variety of torsional parameters will be analyzed and presented as graphs. *AMBER4.1/PME* simulations involving the "Hagerman" (1986) sequences $d[G5-\{GA_4T_4C\}_2-C_5]$ and $d[G_5-\{GT_4A_4C\}_2-C_5]$ are presented here to illustrate the process involved in using *MDTC2.0* and *CURVES*. Experimental evidence characterizes the $d[GA_4T_4C]_n$ as having a compressed minor groove and significant curvature. Conversely, $d[GT_4A_4C]_n$ lacks these features. *MDTC* provides utilities to determine RMS, to extract pdb files from *AMBER* trajectory files, and to view the complete set of DNA helicoidal parameters. *CURVES* analysis is capable of returning measures of curvature and groove width, which are critical in comparing experiment to simulation. A web page auxiliary (http://linus.chem.wesleyan.edu/ima/mdinfo.html) has been created which holds a complete set of *MDTC2.0* example scripts, complete output and links to other programs.

1. Introduction. Current molecular dynamics protocols reach into the nanosecond time range and can produce thousands of archived structures. By contrast, the x-ray crystallographer or NMR spectroscopist will have perhaps a dozen structures based on the same data. Hence, simple weight makes the molecular dynamicist's job more difficult. Customarily, parameters are presented as functions of time. Often, such parameters as energy, RMS and temperature can be taken directly from output files of the MD program being used. Other parameters which are inherent to the geometry of the structure at hand require analysis programs.

Regardless of the particular MD analysis program being used, a strong knowledge of the UNIX operating system and some programing skills are critical. Naturally, MD programs run primarily on some variant of UNIX. Hence, simply starting a simulation requires a rudimentary UNIX capabil-

* Chemistry Department, Wesleyan University, Middletown, CT 06459.

ity. MD *out* files are typically in text format but are not directly graphable. Manipulation of text files thus becomes a critical step in processing data. UNIX provides a variety of utilities for processing text files easily and quickly. The UNIX utilities *sed, nawk, grep, cut* and *paste* can minimize the need to write filter programs in C or Fortran. These utilities are particularly useful for extracting parameters from output files and assembling the output into formats suitable for a graphing package. In recent years, there has been a surge in the use of the freeware PERL programing language since it can combine the easy text manipulation capabilities of the UNIX utilities (*sed, nawk, grep* and others) within a programing language which allows actual calculations to be performed. The web page auxiliary has links to PERL sites.

However, not every desired parameter can be collected from an output file. At this point, a researcher must turn to one or a combination of (1) in-house conveniences, (2) analysis programs inherent to the modeling package he is using or (3) one of the few programs made and distributed specifically for analysis. Animation of MD trajectories is a common example of in-house conveniences as there are currently few standardized ways of porting trajectory files into such packages as Tripos' (St. Louis) *Sybyl* or MSI's (San Diego) *Discover* to create animation. The *CARNAL* (Ross, 1995) program is an example of an analysis program inherent to a specific modeling package. There are several programs intended for analysis of pdb structures for both proteins and DNA.

DNA or RNA analysis revolves around several geometric properties defined relative to the helix axis (helicoidals). An EMBO workshop (Dickerson et al., 1989) gave standard definitions for the helicoidal parameters. Two helicoidals of specific interest are x- displacement and inclination. These are the parameters which differentiate the A- and B- forms of DNA (Fig. 1). Basepairs in A-DNA are slanted (inclined) while B-DNA basepairs are flat relative to the helix axis. A-DNA's characteristic gun barrel appearance comes from significant x-displacement which B-DNA lacks. In addition to the helicoidals, there are several torsions associated with the phosphoribose or phosphodeoxyribose backbone and the pucker (Saenger, 1983). Pucker reflects ribose or deoxyribose ring isomerization which are equivalent to the chair-boat isomerizations seen for six-member rings. A-DNA has a $C3'$-endo pucker (13°) while B-DNA's is $C2'$-endo (154°). In the DNA analysis field, there are several programs which return helicoidal parameters including *NewHelix* (Fratini *et al.*, 1982), CURVES (Lavery and Sklenar, 1996), RNA (Babcock et al. 1994); NUPARM (Bansal *et al.*, 1995) and NAMOT (Soumpasis et al. 1991). A review and analysis of the merits of the various programs by Elgavish and Harvey (1997) concluded that the RNA program and the *CURVES* program were the most reliable. The helix axis for the *CURVES* program can be a global or local smoothly curving construct. *RNA* is based on a local helix axis construct. For both, the helix axis is determined within the programs according to rigorous mathematical definitions. This is in contrast to other programs in which the helix axis must be defined by the user. Both of these programs will return the same set of helicoidals for a structure regardless of which strand is specified as the reading strand. Neither of these programs is intended for direct analysis of MD trajectories.

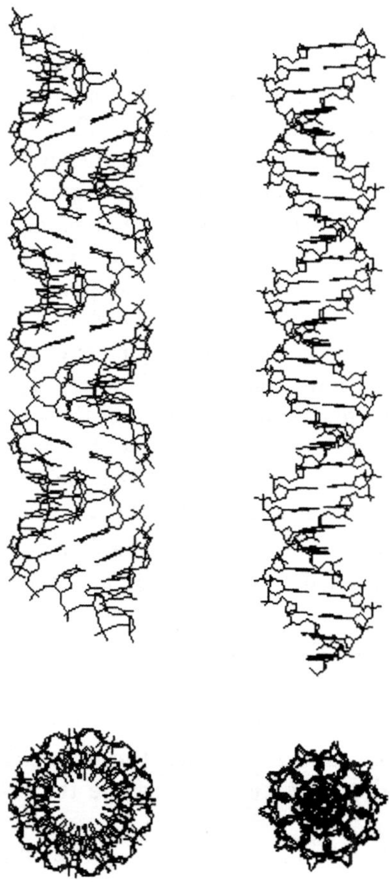

FIG. 1. *The A- and B- forms of DNA for the 30mer sequence* $d[G_5-\{GA_4T_4C\}_2-C_5]$. **Left:** *A-DNA is characterized by inclined basepairs (the slanted appearance) and a significant x-displacement (the hollow helix).* **Right:** *B-DNA has essentially a* 0° *inclination and no significant x-displacement.*

The *Molecular Dynamics ToolChest* (MDTC) suite of programs is one of the few programs which is intended for direct analysis of MD trajectories (Ravishanker and Beveridge, 1996). For DNA analysis, its flagship utility *dials_and_windows_dna* serves as a front end for passing *GROMOS*, *AMBER* or *CHARMm* trajectory files to the *CURVES* program. For proteins, the program *dials_and_windows_proteins* will pass coordinates to CURVES. The program will calculate the common torsions ϕ, ψ, ω and various χ as well as additional geometric measures specific to α-helices and β-sheets (Sklenar *et al.*, 1989; Swaminathan *et al.*, 1990). Time series for all the helicoidal parameters or torsions are then available for graphing.

This paper will concentrate on a walk-through analysis using $MDTC2.0$ for two DNA system examples. The systems simulated are the sequences $d[G_5 - \{GA_4T_4C\}_2 - C_5]$ and $d[G_5 - \{GT_4A_4C\}_2 - C_5]$. While these sequences are identical in content, the change in the polarity of the central $d[A_4T_4]$ subsequence to $d[T_4A_4]$ has dramatic experimental repercussions (Berkhoff and Tullius, 1988; Hagerman, 1986). Figures presented show exactly how raw output from $MDTC2.0$ currently appears. Specifically, $MDTC2.0$ will be used to provide information which is detailed in terms of both structure and time. The maximum resolution for time matches the frequency that structures were archived. Structural maximum resolution is at the parameter definition level. With proteins, for instance, standardized figures presenting ϕ/ψ as functions of time for each amino acid are created. With DNA, standardized figures presenting the various backbone torsion as functions of time for each nucleotide are created. While it would be untrue to claim that $MDTC2.0$ is easy to use the first time, routine use does allow for facile validation of the MD run. This paper has four aims. The first two are concerned with presenting the quality and form of the simulated DNA structures in a concise and easily understood method. These aims exploit current $MDTC2.0$ functionality:

(1) to demonstrate DNA simulation quality at the the maximum resolution possible - nucleotide by nucleotide and time point by time point; and

(2) to demonstrate DNA simulation quality at a global resolution.

The last two aims require functionalities inherent to the CURVES program which are not currently accessed by $MDTC2.0$ directly:

(3) determine the extent to which the $d[GA_4T_4C]$ subsequence simulated in AMBER produces curvature while the$d[GT_4A_4C]$ subsequence does not; and

(4) determine the extent to which the $d[GA_4T_4C]$ subsequence simulated in AMBER has a stable compressed minor groove while the $d[GT_4A_4C]$ subsequence does not.

These results agree with the experiments of Hagerman (1986) and Berkhoff and Tullius (1988). We stress, however, that these example cases are preliminary.

This paper is inherently transient and will be outdated within a few years. We have created a web page (http://linus.chem.wesleyan.edu/ima/mdinfo.html) which will provide example scripts, complete output and links to internet documentation. It is recognized that internet web pages are fluid and subjected to only the friendliest of peer review. However, access to complete example scripts which can be downloaded and modified can save hours or days of work. Hence, we feel it is appropriate to include.

2. Molecular Dynamics ToolChest applied to the Hagerman sequences.

Overview of the MDTC2.0 programs . Fig. 2 shows a flow chart for analysis with the *MDTC*2.0 program suite. Trajectories are pre-processed by removing waters. This is done to make more manageably sized files. While this is not an absolute requirement, it does make additional work much faster. Counterions and small bound ligands are typically not significant contributors to file size as compared to the DNA itself. Hence, there is less motive to remove these. After this pre- processing, a variety of programs can read the trajectories and perform analysis. Aside from *dials_and_windows_dna*, there are the programs *rms, dccm, solvent_accessibility* and *extract_coordinates* (see web page for example scripts).

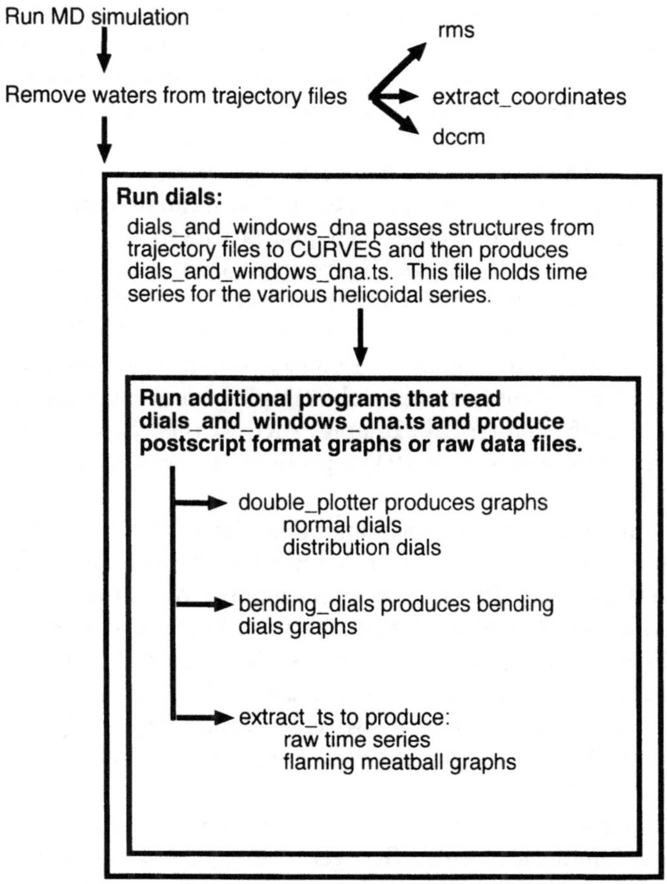

FIG. 2. *Flow chart for MDTC2.0 analysis.*

Executing *extract_coordinates* and producing a few pdb files is a good idea. This is not advocated for the simple extraction of structures to pdb format. Invariably, MD packages will have a utility to do this more efficiently. *Extract_coordinates* use is advocated as a trouble shooting method. If there has been an error in processing the trajectory files - for example, the trajectory files have box dimensions and the user failed to set the correct *MDTC2.0* variable to specify this - then the visual inspection will quickly reveal something is wrong. Since numbering and ordering errors are cumulative, if something in the processing of the trajectories is amiss, the first structures pulled from the trajectory files would be reasonable while the last structures would be sterically impossible. Since scripts used with *extract_coordinates* will be nearly identical to those for the other programs, this first script can be modified quickly for execution of additional commands.

There are several programs which read trajectories directly. The *rms*, *dccm* and *dials_and_windows_dna* programs are discussed here. The program *rms* has two main functions. The first is a simple calculation of RMS versus a reference structure. This leads to the simple and common presentation of RMS as a function of time for the simulation. The second calculation leads to a 2D RMS plot (McConnell *et al.*, 1994). This is a contour plot. The shading at some point represents the RMS between two structures in the simulation, not between the simulated structure at some particular time and a reference. This plot is a method of recognizing substates (McConnell *et al.*, 1994). The program *dccm* allows the creation of a "dynamical cross-correlation map" (Swaminathan *et al.*, 1991). This type of study is useful in protein structures, and potentially for RNA structures. The study will identify regions of a molecule that have correlated motions. Naturally, it will identify the trivial example of sequential amino acids. It will also identify non-trivial examples such as the "flap", "fulcrum" and "cantilever" motions seen in HIV-1 protease dimer MD (Swaminathan *et al.*, 1991).

The program *dials_and_windows_dna* allows the calculation of helicoidals for every structure in a trajectory file. It reads in a reference pdb and trajectory files. The sequence and number of atoms in the reference pdb must match that of the trajectory files. These coordinates are passed to the *CURVES* program. All helicoidals are recorded as time series and deposited in a binary file dials_and_windows.ts. This file is referenced by additional utilities which produce postscript format figures. Currently, there are three utilities which read the dials_and_windows.ts file: *double_plotter, bending_dials and extract_ts.*

Double_plotter produces standardized graphs. The backbone torsions follow the definition given in Saenger (1983) and are presented as polar graphs. North is 0° and torsions progress clockwise. The radius is the time axis, the center being time zero and the outer edge being the end of the simulation (Fig. 3). Distribution dials can also be produced (Fig. 4). These are identical to those previously discussed, except for the addition of an outer irregular line which is proportional to the population at a given angle. All the basepair helicoidals are presented as rectangular graphs. In these, time is simply the vertical axis. Output is in postscript format.

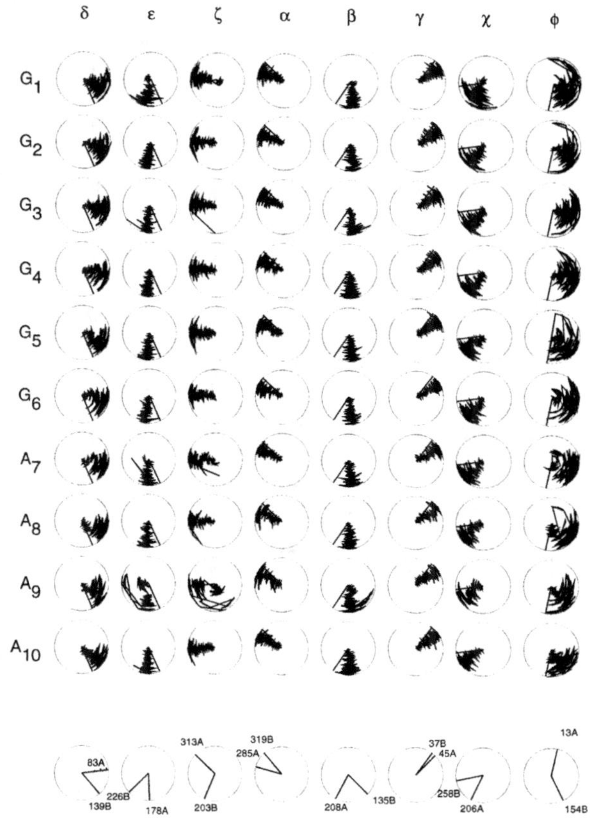

FIG. 3. *Sample output from double_plotter. Greek letters refer to the backbone torsion as defined in Saenger (1983). Roman letters refer to the first 10 nucleotides for the example case sequence* $d[G_4 - \{GA_4T_4C\}_2 - C_5]$. *Each dial is a polar graph where radius is time and* $0°$ *points north. Time ranges from 0 at the center to 1100 ps at the edge. Torsion angles increase in a clockwise manner. The heavy line in each dials is the value of the parameter at time zero. For this simulation, the structure started at canonical B- DNA as produced by the AMBER utility NUCGEN so all nucleotides have the same backbone torsions at time zero. Bottom set of dials presents reference A- and B-DNA values. This is the first page (note "page 0" at bottom) of 21 postscript format images (all are available at web page).*

DNA curvature is typically described in terms of successive roll and tilt deflections (Bolshoy *et al.*, 1991; Zhurkin, 1985). *Bending_dials* presents curvature information for each dinucleotide step as a polar scatter plot. *Bending_dials* follows a convention established earlier (Olson *et al.*, 1988; Zhurkin, 1985) of presenting local DNA curvature on a dinucleotide step by

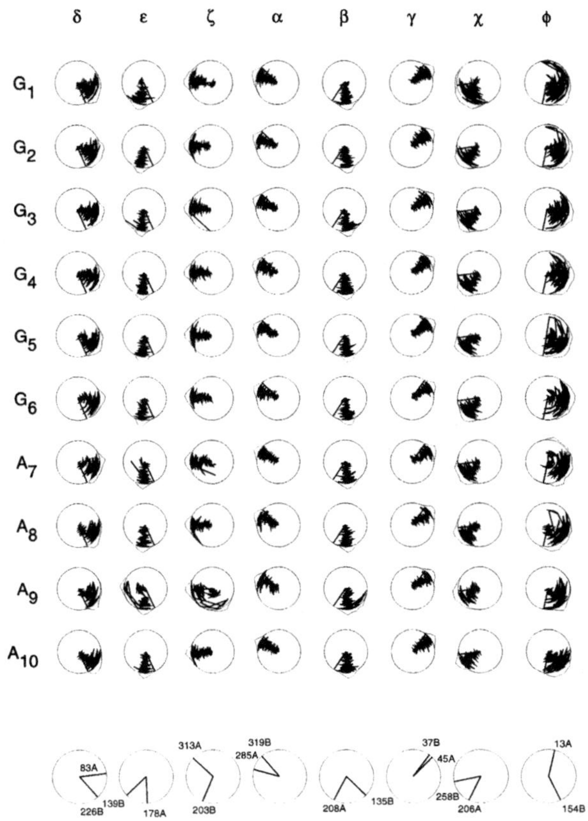

FIG. 4. *Same plot as seen in Fig. 2 but the distribution option is set to true (see web page example script). Population at a given angle is proportional to the "hump" on the dial.*

step basis in terms of a total bending magnitude and an orientation angle. The relation between measured roll (ρ) and tilt (τ) and bending magnitude (θ) and direction (ϕ) is (Young *et al.*, 1995):

$$\theta = [\rho^2 + \tau^2]^{1/2}$$

The direction is defined by these equations:

$$\begin{aligned}
&\text{if } \rho > 0: \\
&\qquad \phi = \arctan(\tau/\rho) \qquad\qquad \text{if } \tau > 0 \\
&\qquad \phi = 360 + \arctan(\tau/\rho) \qquad \text{if } \tau < 0 \\
&\text{if } \rho < 0: \\
&\qquad \phi = 180 + \arctan(\tau/\rho)
\end{aligned}$$

In the polar graph, henceforce called a bending dial, θ is the radius and ϕ is the angle. North on such a plot is the major groove and south is the minor groove. The strand which lies to the left of the dial runs 5′ to 3′. Fig. 5 presents some *bending_dials* output for a segment of the $d[G_5 - \{GA_4T_4C\}_2 - C_5]$ sequence.

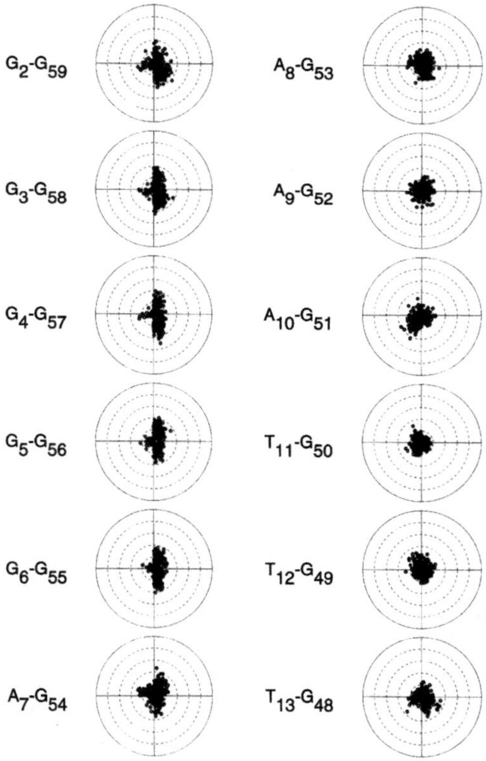

FIG. 5. *Sample bending_dials output. See text for definition of radius and angle. This is the first of three pages of output generated by bending_dials for a 30mer (note "page 0").*

Extract_ts currently performs two duties. It produces the "flaming meatball" distribution dials for the whole trajectory (Fig. 6) and also produces raw time series for all of the torsions and helicoidals in text format. The "flaming meatball" distribution dials are presented on a single page. All the backbone torsions and the pucker are presented for all nucleotides, all purines, all pyrimidines and the four bases. This figure provides a succinct representation of the DNA form that the backbone torsions adopt. The raw time series are simply a group of files which hold values for a particular helicoidal or torsion as time series. These can be subjected to analysis or graphed.

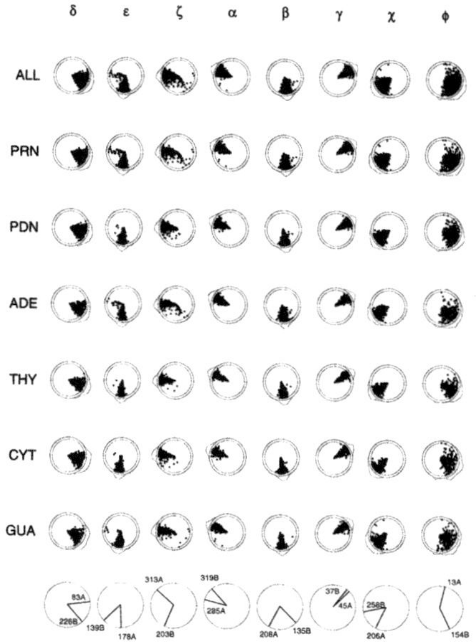

FIG. 6. *Sample output from extract_ts. This is similar to the output in Fig 2. A key difference is that it is organized by pooling the torsions into seven bins: ALL, all torsions for every nucleotide in the sequence; PRN: all torsions for the purines; PDN: all torsions for the pyrimidines; and a pooling for each of the bases. This provides an easily inspected figure to see the form of the DNA.*

3. Example case: the Hagerman sequences $d[G5-\{GA_4T_4C\}_2-C_5]$ **and** $d[G_5-\{GT_4A_4C\}_2-C_5]$. The B-DNA helix has roughly 10.5 basepairs per helix turn (Saenger, 1983). Hence, sequences of the form $d[A_iX_k]_n$, where $i+k$ is roughly 10 and i is 4 to 6, are called phased A-tracts since the A-tract is in phase with the helix repeat. Marini et *al.* (1982) observed that sequences of this form obtained from trypanosomes (a eukaryote which causes sleeping sickness in man and cattle) migrated anomalously slowly on polyacrylamide gels. This gel anomaly was postulated to originate from inherent curvature in the sequences. Hagerman (1984) demonstrated that the same sequence motif would produce a shorter than expected electric birefringence decay constant. This result is consistent with a more compact structure originating from curvature. Cyclization studies look at the balance between circles formed and concatamers formed in the presence of DNA ligase. Here, if the DNA is highly curved, a greater population of circles is expected. Ulanovsky *et al.* (1986) demonstrated this phenomenon. In short, the early postulation that gel anomaly is a function of curvature has been supported by additional methods. Hagerman (1990) provides an excellent review of the key experiments done during the 1980s in this field. However, it is diffucult to translate solution structure measurements into atomic level or even basepair level models. Hence, crystal structures providing atomic resolution were eagerly awaited.

Unfortunately, crystal structures of A-tracts have provided a contradictory image that A- tracts are straight (DiGabriele *et al.*, 1989; DiGabriele and Steitz, 1993; Goodsell *et al.*, 1993; Grzeskowiak *et al.*, 1993; Nelson *et al.*, 1987). Making the assumption that G-rich general sequence DNA is curved and that A-tracts bring their curvature into phase can explain a good deal of gel anomaly, cyclization and other solution structure measurement data (Goodsell *et al.*, 1993; Grzeskowiak *et al.*, 1993). However, there are some problem sequences. Specifically, the sequences studied by Hagerman (1986) are difficult to explain in terms of a curved G-rich general sequence model. Why would $d[CA_4T_4G]_n$ and $d[GA_4T_4C]_n$ be curved while $d[CT_4A_4G]_n$ and $d[GT_4A_4C]_n$ not be curved if the curvature lies in the guanine-cytosine basepairs?

The discrepancies between solution structure measurements and crystallography are reconciled when solution structure measurements are taken under conditions which more closely match the crystal milieu. It has been recently demonstrated by several independent experiments that 2-methyl-2,4-pentanediol (MPD) - used to induce DNA crystallization - reduces A-tract curvature. Sprous *et al.* (1995), inspired by earlier studies which demonstrated that ethanol straightens A-tracts (Marini *et al.*, 1984), observed that MPD reduced gel anomalies. Additional studies showed that the characteristic signals of curvature were reduced in electron microscopy and cyclization studies as MPD concentrations were raised (Dlakic *et al.*, 1996; Harvey *et al.*, 1995). Chemical probing of A-tracts likewise demonstrated that the structure changes with MPD present (Ganunis *et al.*, 1996). MPD's effect is specific to A-tracts and the phenomenon should not be extrapolated to dismiss all DNA crystal curvature measurements. Indeed, dodecamers holding the subsequence $d[G_2C_2]$ have been seen in crystal to show notable curvature (Goodsell *et al.*, 1993). Closely related sequences of the form $d[XXG_3C_3XX]_n$ will exhibit gel anomalies and cyclization patterns characteristic of curved DNA independent of MPD concentration (Brukner *et al.*, 1994; Dlakic *et al.*, 1996). However, the experimental evidence strongly supports the conclusion that A-tracts are straightened by MPD (Dlakic *et al.*, 1996; Ganunis *et al.*, 1996; Harvey *et al.*, 1995; Sprous *et al.*, 1995). Extrapolation from A-tract structure observed under the influence of MPD to A-tract structure under more physiological conditions should be done with caution and cross- referencing to other methodologies for verification is crucial. The questions concerning A- tract crystal structure and the limited resolution of solution measurements does provide an added motive for modeling A-tracts.

For our simulation, there are two critical experiments. First, Hagerman (1986) showed that the $d[A_4T_4]$ motif is curved while the $d[T_4A_4]$ motif is straight. Second, Tullius and coworkers (Berkhoff and Tullius, 1988) demonstrated that the $d[A_4T_4]$ motif exhibits a distinctive hydroxyl radical cleavage pattern while the $d[T_4A_4]$ motif does not. This cleavage pattern has been interpreted as evidence for a compressed minor groove. Ideally, we hope to provide atomic resolution models for the A-tract curvature phenomenon. Such models would strongly complement the low resolution solution structure data. To attack the A-tract structure issue, we modeled the sequences $d[G_5 - \{GA_4T_4C\}_2 - C_5]$ and $d[G_5 - \{GT_4A_4C\}_2 - C_5]$ using the *AMBER4.1* package (Cornell *et al.*, 1995; Pearlman *et al.*, 1995). The Young *et al.* (1997) paper presents the minimization, heating, equilibration and production dynamics methodology. The most interesting questions in simulating the sequences $d[G_5 - \{GA_4T_4C\}_2 - C_5]$ and $d[G_5 - \{GT_4A_4C\}_2 - C_5]$ are: "Is $d[G_5 - \{GA_4T_4C\}_2 - C_5]$ curved and is $d[G_5 - \{GT_4A_4C\}_2 - C_5]$ straight under appropriate conditions?" and Is a compressed minor groove observable in the $d[G_5 - GA_4T_4C_2 - C_5]$ sequence?". The basic questions in simulating the two sequences are more mundane and critical: "Are these structures in the B-DNA structure family?", "Is the structure reasonable or is it unwinding?" and "Is the simulation converged enough to answer the interesting questions?". Obviously, the data taken directly from the MD output file will not provide answers to either the interesting nor the basic questions.

The first stage in *MDTC2.0* analysis is to remove the waters, counterions and ligands. This will make for more manageable files as was discussed above. *Extract_coordinates* is then run to confirm that the processing has gone smoothly to this point (see web page for example). *RMS* was run to produce a fairly ordinary plot of RMS(t) (not shown here, see web page for example script and plot).

To address whether the trajectory is structurally valid, we executed *dials_and_windows_dna* as a first step in producing graphs of all the helicoidal parameters. The web page presents example scripts. We then executed *double_plotter* to produce the full set of plots for the helicoidal parameters. For this system with 30 basepairs and the *MDTC2.0* variable "number_of_rows" set to 10, *double_plotter* requires 21 pages to present all the torsions and helicoidals. This is obviously not something that would be published normally and is not presented in print with this chapter. However, it is quite useful to monitor the quality of the simulation.

Fig. 3 is the first of six pages (see web page for additional 5) of figures which present torsion and pucker dials. The structural resolution of these figures is at the nucleotide level. The maximum time resolution is limited only by the frequency that structures were archived. Each dial is a polar graph which presents for a given torsion of a given nucleotide that torsion as a function of time. The standardized figures also define the starting structure and the canonical values accepted for $A-$ and $B-$ DNA. Inspection of these figures shows that pucker is in the $B - DNA$ range. Fig. 4 provides much the same information as Fig. 3. The outer irregular line is proportional to the population at a given angle. Hence, Fig. 4 is a distribution graph as well as a simple time series. Simple rectangular graphs are provided for the translational and rotational helicoidals (see web page). Inspection of these graphs shows that on a nucleotide-by- nucleotide basis, the structure has x-displacement and inclination values associated with $B-DNA$. The simplest method to demonstrate global $B-DNA$ character is to pool the torsions and plot them as a distribution dial. *Extract_ts* does this to produce the figure seen in Fig. 6. Here, the torsions are pooled into bins for all nucleotides, all purine nucleotide, all pyrimidine nucleotides and a pool for each base. Again, the data points to a $B - DNA$ conformation. On the whole, the trajectories are well-behaved and the structures are reasonable for $B - DNA$. This data is for the $d[G_5 - \{GA_4T_4C\}_2 - C_5]$ sequence. The raw output for the $d[G_5 - \{GT_4A_4C\}_2 - C_5]$ sequence is available at the web page.

We executed *bending_dials* to provide information concerning local curvature (see Fig. 5 and web page) on a dinucleotide step by dinucleotide step basis. Since the two structures shown in Fig. 7 are fairly typical for their respective trajectories, one would expect an easily interpretable set of bending dials for each trajectory. Specifically, the exact loci of bending should be obvious for the $d[G_5 - \{GA_4T_4C\}_2 - C_5]$ sequence. It is difficult to find such information by simple visual inspection. Identifying the exact loci of curvature for this system will require more work and analysis than simply looking at parameters based on roll and tilt. When we determine what is required, a new *MDTC2.0* utility will be developed to make its extraction easier.

In short, *MDTC2.0* allowed a facile determination of DNA form on a nucleotide-by-nucleotide basis and at a global resolution across all simulated time. More than that, the concise bending dials and distribution dials put the information in a format which was comprehensible by simple visual inspection. The distribution dials for the $d[G_5 - \{GA_4T_4C\}_2 - C_5]$ sequence (complete set available at the web page) and for the $d[G_5 - \{GT_4A_4C\}_2 - C_5]$ sequence (not shown) provide easily comprehensible proof that the structure is in the $B - DNA$ family. A detailed review of the output helicoidals shows that there are no gross irregularities (the output from *double_plotter* is available at the web page for inspection). Further, the parameters are oscillating within definable regions of conformational space. Though convergence can never be unquestionably established, stability within a defined region of conformational space is a minimum requirement for a converged trajectory. The important questions to ask of the trajectories (i.e., are these structures reasonable) are answered favorably.

The interesting questions can be addressed with a greater level of confidence since it is now established that conclusions will not based on conformationally unreasonable structures. The key questions are whether the $d[G_5 - \{GA_4T_4C\}_2 - C_5]$ sequence is curved and whether the $d[G_5 - \{GT_4A_4C\}_2 - C_5]$ is straight. Ideally, this would be revealed by analysis of roll and tilt. However, the bending dials are difficult to interpret. Simple

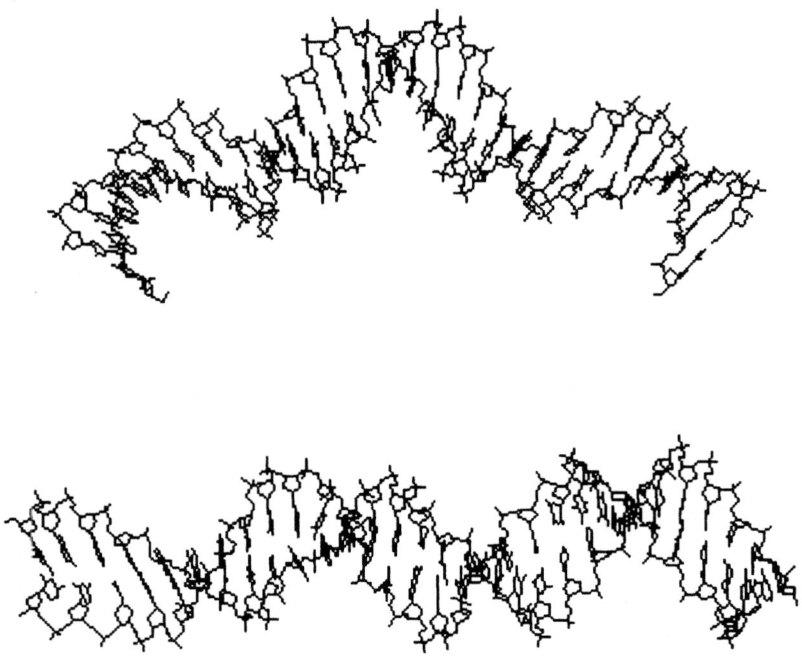

FIG. 7. *Wireframe images of typical structures from the two trajectories. These images were produced by RasMol.* **Top**: *the* 950 *ps structure for the* $d[G_4 - \{GA_4T_4C\}_2 - C_5]$ *sequence.* **Bottom**: *the* 950 *ps structure for the* $d[G_4 - \{GT_4A_4C\}_2 - C_5]$ *sequence.*

wireframe images suggest that the $d[G_5 - \{GA_4T_4C\}_2 - C_5]$ sequence is curved and the $d[G_5 - \{GT_4A_4C\}_2 - C_5]$ is normally straight (see Fig. 7). Identifying where this curvature arises in the bending dials presentations of roll/tilt is difficult and unclear. Further, *MDTC2.0* does not currently provide gross measures of curvature as a function of time nor does it present a rigorous measure of groove width, a parameter of interest in light of Berkhoff and Tullius (1988). To produce gross measures of curvature and groove width measurements, *CURVES* must be used directly.

4. Direct application of CURVES to the "Hagerman" sequences. Visual inspection of the structures leads to the conclusion that for most of the length of the two trajectories, $d[G_5 - \{GA_4T_4C\}_2 - C_5]$ is curved and $d[G_5 - \{GT_4A_4C\}_2 - C_5]$ is straight (Fig. 7). However, presenting several hundred structures is not practical for any publication. In the future as web auxiliaries for journals become more robust and accepted, perhaps a web-based animation would help present the nature of these two simulations. However, in the interim, a simple gross curvature as a function of time is needed. Simple measurements based on end-to-end distance of the segments and deflection angle should confirm or deny the interpretation of visual inspection. *CURVES* provided two measurements which are useful for gross curvature: shortening and total curvature angle. Shortening is defined below:

$$\text{shortening} = (1 - L)/1$$

where L is the end-to-end distance and l is the contour length. Contour length is the length of the DNA segment if one were to move a probe along it like a roadway. End-to-end distance is the through space distance between the first and last basepairs. The total curvature angle is defined as the angle between the first and last dyad axis segments. *CURVES* also provides a measure of the groove widths and depths (Boutonnet *et al.*, 1993; Stofer and Lavery, 1993). As already mentioned, *CURVES* is not designed to analyze MD trajectories directly.

The web page provides an example script for passing structures from an MD trajectory to *CURVES* and extracting shortening, curvature angle and minor groove width. It uses the *MDTC2.0* utility *extract_coordinates* to pull pdb files from the trajectory files. These are passed to *CURVES*. The UNIX utility *grep* is used to directly select and record the text line holding the shortening and the curvature angle. The format for the minor groove width is too irregular to be processed by invoking *grep*. A *gawk* (GNU variant of the UNIX utility *awk*) script is required to help produce the file minor.dat which holds for each basepair an entry recording the minor groove width at a particular timepoint. The minor groove entries are subjected to analysis later. This was repeated for every 100 ps block.

The graphs in Fig. 8 presents shortening and curvature angle as functions of time for the two Hagerman sequences. The greater curvature of the $d[G_5 - \{GA_4T_4C\}_2 - C_5]$ sequence relative the $d[G_5 - \{GT_4A_4C\}_2 - C_5]$ sequence is easily seen. The web page presents the complete set of 100 ps averages for the minor groove analysis. By looking at the minor groove profiles on a 100 ps block by 100 ps block basis, we saw a single characteristic pattern for the $d[G_5 - \{GA_4T_4C\}_2 - C_5]$ sequence and three distinct pattern types for the $d[G_5 - \{GT_4A_4C\}_2 - C_5]$ sequence. The three substate groove width patterns as well as typical groove width patterns for the $d[G_5 - \{GA_4T_4C\}_2 - C_5]$ sequence are presented in Fig 9. Specifically, the two $d[A_4T_4]$ motifs always have minor groove minima near the center of the motif. There is a maximum at the center of the central $d[T_4CGA_4]$ section. The three distinct patterns in the $d[G_5 - \{GT_4A_4C\}_2 - C_5]$ sequence are (1) from 0 – 100 ps, compressed minor groove in the flanking regions, (2) from 200 – 400 ps, a pattern near identical to that described for the $d[G_5 - \{GA_4T_4C\}_2 - C_5]$ sequence, and (3) from 400 – 1200 ps, multiple minima and maxima with no firm location. It is possible that the two early appearing substates are part of a long equilibration process. The minor groove compression pattern seen for the $d[G_5 - \{GA_4T_4C\}_2 - C_5]$ sequence and for the dominant substate for the $d[G_5 - \{GT_4A_4C\}2 - C_5]$ sequence agrees well with the experiments of Tullius and coworkers (Berkhoff

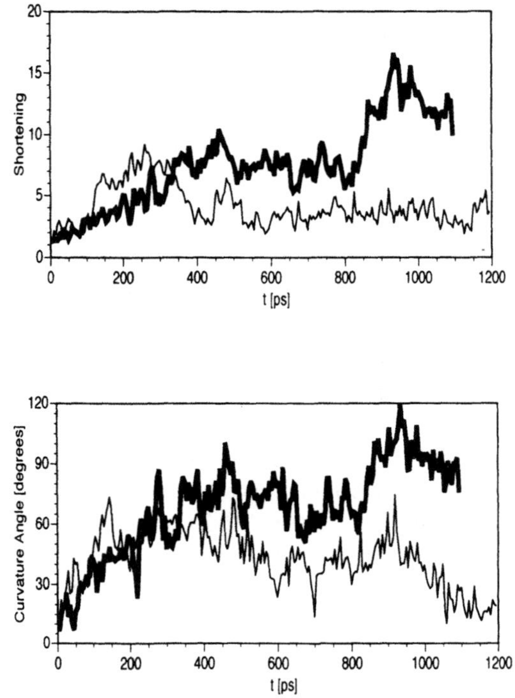

FIG. 8. *Top: Shortening as a function of time for the two trajectories. Bottom: curvature angle as a function of time for the two trajectories.* $d[G_4 - \{GA_4T_4C\}_2 - C_5]$ *is shown by a thick line and* $d[G_4 - \{GT_4A_4C\}_2 - C_5]$ *by a thin line.*

and Tullius, 1988; Ganunis *et al.*, 1996). Curvature, as observed visually and in the plots of shortening and curvature angle, is weak in the dominant substate for the $d[G_5 - \{GT_4A_4C\}_2 - C_5]$ sequence.

Analysis by *MDTC2.0* and *CURVES* suggests that *AMBER4.1* produces excellent structures when compared to experiment. The values of the various helicoidals and backbone torsions are close to B-DNA canonical. Sequence specific curvature (Hagerman, 1986) and groove width patterns (Berkhoff and Tullius, 1987; Ganunis *et al.*, 1996) agree with solution structure measurements. These trajectories provide atomic resolution models for solution A-tract structure - a phenomenon almost entirely defined by such low resolution methods such as gel anomaly, cyclization and electric birefringence.

5. Other analysis resources: Protein analysis and visual presentations. There are numerous protein analysis tools. Few are really meant for analysis of MD- trajectories. *MDTC2.0*, as already mentioned, will provide some analysis for proteins. The *Discover-Decipher* module can analyze protein trajectories, provided that they are put in a format that *Discover* can read. There are a variety of programs intended to test whether

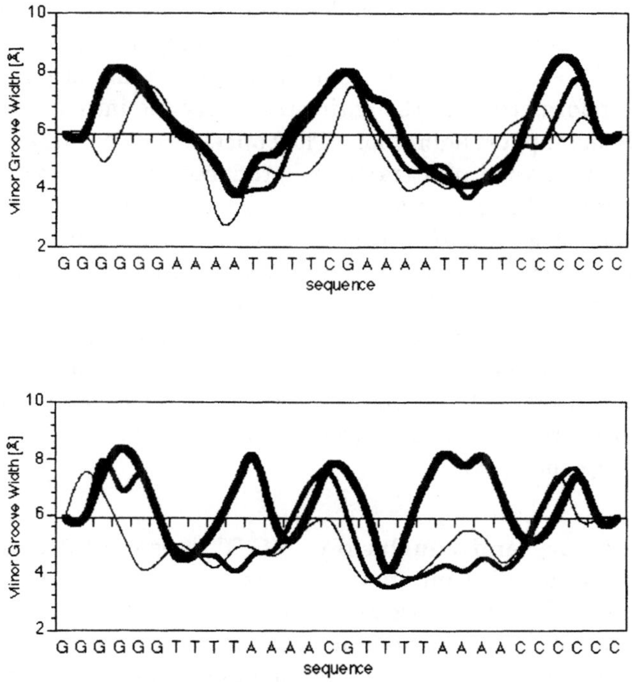

FIG. 9. *Minor groove width as a function of sequence. Top: for the* d$[G_4 - \{GA_4T_4C\}_2 - C_5]$ *sequence, thickest line is the average for 1000-1100 ps, thinner line is for 0-100 ps and thinnest line is for 600-700 ps. Bottom: for the* d$[G_4 - \{GT_4A_4C\}_2 - C_5]$ *sequence, thickest line is the average for 100-200 ps, thinner line is for 200-300 ps and thinnest line is for 500-600 ps. The time ranges selected for the first sequence were chosen more or less at random, the time ranges for the second correspond to recognizable substates. The earlier substates in* d$[G_4 - \{GT_4A_4C\}_2 - C_5]$ *do show curvature while the later does not. Note the simple form of the* d$[G_4 - \{GA_4T_4C\}_2 - C_5]$ *pattern versus the greater variety of the* d$[G_4 - \{GT_4A_4C\}_2 - C_5]$ *pattern. Web page has more complete figures of the minor groove width.*

a protein structure is structurally reasonable or to determine secondary structural motifs. Kabsch and Sander (1983) presented an algorithm for determining secondary structure based on pattern recognition of hydrogen bonds and geometric features. This algorithm has been incorporated into other classification programs. Other methodologies include the 3D profiles developed by Luthy *et al.* (1992), protein shape comparison (Holm and Sander, 1996), solvation free energy analysis (Eisenberg and McLachlan, 1986) and graphical representations of hydrogen bonding patterns in proteins (Factor and Mehler, 1991). These methods could be potentially adapted to analysis of protein trajectories or to average structures from MD.

There are a large number of programs available for visual presentations of molecular structures. Programs such as *Quanta* (MSI, San Diego) and

Sybyl (Tripos, St. Louis) are complete modeling packages. Direct reading of trajectory files from competitors programs is highly variable. Typically, extraction of a single structure from the trajectory file in pdb format or a complete reformatting of the entire trajectory file into a new format is required. Some support animation. They operate only on workstation class computers. Animation of a trajectory produced within these packages is relatively simple. Porting in a trajectory from another modeling package, such as porting in an *AMBER* trajectory into *Discover*, requires an in-house filter program to change formats. The freeware *Visual Molecular Dynamics* (VMD) program developed by Schulten and coworkers (Humphrey *et al.*, 1996) operates on SGI computers. The program is reported to be capable of reading a large variety input file types and producing animation. Creation of animation readable by webbrowsers such as Netscape is also possible. The examples presented to date (see web page for links) do not allow the user to change the view.

6. Summary and conclusion. *MDTC2.0* is currently tuned to return exact and detailed information concerning the form of a simulated DNA sequence. Its routine use allows the facile description of DNA structure in terms of form. Structural resolution is at the definition of the parameter on a nucleotide- by-nucleotide basis. Time resolution is limited only by the frequency that structures are archived. It can also provide global information that is easily interpreted in terms of form. Currently, the program does not provide critical global parameters such as shortening and gross curvature angle. These will be incorporated into the program in the near future.

The simulations presented are important scientifically since they demonstrate that AMBER4.1 can match key experimental properties of phased A-tract structure. Specifically, we see B-DNA structure persisting into the nanosecond time domain. Cheatham and Kollman (1996) had earlier seen this for decamer sequences. More importantly, AMBER4.1 is able to reproduce curvature and a compressed minor groove for the $d[G_5 - \{GA_4T_4C\}_2 - C_5]$ sequence with no additional constraints while at the same time not showing these same traits for the $d[G_5 - \{GT_4A_4C\}_2 - C_5]$ sequence. These results match experimental measures (Berkhoff and Tullius, 1988; Hagerman, 1986) and are surprising successes.

Acknowledgments: NIGMS award GM-37909 to Dr. D.L. Beveridge supported this work. G. Ravishanker is the principle author of *MDTC2.0*. W. Wang is currently debuging and adding enhancements to the program suite. D. Sprous in close collaboration with M.A. Young (Wesleyan University) performed the described simulations on the PSC's T3D and on the NCSA's Power Challenge Array. The author thanks Joy McConnell for editorial help.

REFERENCES

[1] Babcock, M. S., E. P. D. Pednault, and W. K. Olson. 1994. Nucleic acid structure analysis. J. Mol. Biol. 237:125–156

[2] Bansal-M, Bhattacharyya-D, and Ravi-B. 1995. NUPARM and NUCGEN: software for analysis and generation of sequence dependent nucleic acid structures. Comput-Appl-Biosci 11:281–287.

[3] Berkhoff, A. M., and T. D. Tullius. 1988. Structural details of an adenine tract that does not cause DNA to bend. Nature 331:455–456.

[4] Bolshoy, A., P. McNamara, R. E. Harrington, and E. N. Trifonov. 1991. Curved DNA without A-A: experimental estimation of all 16 DNA wedge angles. Proc. Natl. Acad. Sci. USA 88:2313–2316.

[5] Boutonnet, N., X. Hui, and K. Zakrzewska. 1993. Looking into the grooves of DNA. Biopolymers 33:479–490.

[6] Breslauer, K. J. 1991. A Thermodynamic perspective of DNA bending. Curr. Opin. Struct. Bio. 1:416–422.

[7] Chan, S. C., K. J. Breslauer, M. E. Hogan, D. J. Kessler, R. H. Austin, J. Ojemann, J. M. Passner, and N. C. Wiles. 1990. Physical studies of DNA premelting equilibria in duplexes with and without homo $dA \cdot dT$ tracts: correlations with DNA bending. Biochemistry 29:6161–6171.

[8] Chan, S. C., K. J. Breslauer, R. H. Austin, and M. E. Hogan. 1993. Thermodynamics and premelting conformational changes of phased $d(A)5$ tracts. Biochemistry 32:11776–11784.

[9] Cheatham, T. E., and P. A. Kollman. 1996. Observation of the A-DNA to B-DNA transition during unrestrained molecular dynamics in aqueous solution. *J. Mol. Biol.* 259:434–444.

[10] Cornell, W. D., P. Cieplak, C. I. Bayly, I. R. Gould, K. M. Merz, D. M. Fergusin, D. C. Spellmeyer, T. Fox, J. W. Caldwell, and P. A. Kollman. 1995. A second generation force field for the simulation of proteins, nucleic acids and organic molecules. *J. Am. Chem. Soc.* 117:5179–5197.

[11] Dickerson, R. E., M. Bansal, C. R. Calladine, S. Diekman, W. N. Hunter, O. Kennard, E. von Kitzing, R. Lavery, H. C. M. Nelson, W. K. Olson, W. Saenger, Z. Shakked, H. Skenar, D. M. Soumpasis, C. S. Tung, A. H. J. Wang, and V. B. Zhurkin. 1989. Definition and nomenclature of nucleic acid structural parameters. *EMBO* J. 8:1–4.

[12] DiGabriele, A. D., M. R. Sanderson, and T. A. Steitz. 1989. Crystal lattice packing is important in determining the bend of a DNA dodecamer containing an adenine tract. *Proc. Natl. Acad. Sci.* USA 86:1816–1820.

[13] DiGabriele, A. D., and T. A. Steitz. 1993. A DNA dodecamer containing an adenine tract crystallizes in a unique lattice and exhibits a new bend. *J. Mol. Biol.* 231:1024–1039.

[14] Dlakic, M., K. Parks, J. D. Griffith, S. C. Harvey, and R. E. Harrington. 1996. The organic crystallizing agent 2-methyl-2,4-pentanediol reduces DNA curvature by means of structural changes in A-tracts. *J. Biol. Chem.* 271:17911–17919.

[15] Eisenberg, D., and A. D. McLachlan. 1986. Solvation energy in protein folding and binding. *Nature* 319:199–203.

[16] Elgavish, T., and S. C. Harvey. 1997. Comparative analysis of programs that calculate nucleic acid helicoidal parameters. *preprint*

[17] Factor, A. D., and E. L. Mehler. 1991. Graphical representation of hydrogen bonding patterns in proteins. *Protein Eng.* 4:421–425.

[18] Fratini, A. V., M. L. Kopka, H. R. Drew, and R. E. Dickerson. 1982. Reversible bending and helix geometry in a B-DNA dodecamer: CGCGAATT(BrC)GCG. *J. Biol. Chem.* 257:14686–14707.

[19] Ganunis, R., H. Guo, and T. D. Tullius. 1996. Effect of the crystallizing agent 2-methyl-2,4-pentanediol on the structure of adenine tract DNA in solution. *Biochemistry* 35:13729–13732.

[20] Goodsell, D. S., M. L. Kopka, D. Cascio, and R. E. Dickerson. 1993. Crystal structure of CATGGCCATG and its implications for A-Tract bending models. *Proc. Natl. Acad. Sci.* USA 90:2930–2934.

[21] Grzeskowiak, K., D. S. Goodsell, M. Kaczor-Grzeskowiak, D. Cascio, and R. E. Dickerson. 1993. Crystallographic analysis of C-C-A-A-G-C-T- T-G-G and its implications for bending in B-DNA. *Biochemistry* 32:8923–8931.

[22] Hagerman, P. J. 1986. Sequence-directed curvature of DNA. *Nature* 321:449–450.

[23] Hagerman, P. J. 1990. Sequence-directed curvature of DNA. *Annu. Rev. Biochem.* 59:755–781.

[24] Harvey, S. C., M. Dlakic, J. Giffiths, R. E. Harrington, K. Park, D. Sprous, and W. Zacharias. 1995. What is the basis of sequence-directed curvature in DNAs containing A-tracts. *J. Biomolec. Struct. Dyns.* 13:301–307.

[25] Harvey, S. C., M. A. Young, D. Sprous, and D.L. Beveridge. 1997. What does X-ray cystallography teach us about sequence directed curvature. *Proc. Natl. Acad. Sci.* submitted:

[26] Holm, L., and Sander C. 1996. Mapping the protein universe. Science 273:595–602.

[27] Humphrey W., A. Dalke, and K. Schulten. 1996. VMD — Visual Molecular Dynamics. J. Molec. Graphics 14:33–38.

[28] Kabsch, W., and C. Sander. 1983. Dictionary of protein secondary structure: pattern recognition of hydrogen-bonded and geometrical features. Biopolymers 25:2577–2637.

[29] Lavery, R., and H. Sklenar. 1996. CURVES 5.1. CERN, Paris, France

[30] Lüthy, R., J. U. Bowie, and D. Eisenberg. 1992. Assessment of protein models with three-dimensional profiles. Nature 356:83–85.

[31] Marini, J. C., P. N. Effron, T. C. Goodman, C. K. Singleton, R. D. Wells, R. M. Wartell, and P. T. Englund. 1984. Physical characterization of a kinetoplast DNA fragment with unusual properties. J. Biol. Chem. 259:8974–8979.

[32] McConnell, K. J., R. Nirmala, M. A. Young, G. Ravishanker, and D. L. Beveridge. 1994. A nanosecond molecular dynamics trajectory for a BDNA double helix: evidence for substates. J. Am. Chem. Soc. 116:4461–4462.

[33] Nelson, H. C. M., J. T. Finch, B. F. Luisi, and A. Klug. 1987. The structure of an oligo(dA).oligo(dT) yract and its biological implications. Nature 330:221–226.

[34] Olson, W. K., A. R. Srinivasan, M. Hao, and J. L. Nauss. Base sequence dependent models of DNA curvature. 1988. Structure and Expression. 225–242. Adenine Press, Schenectady NY USA.

[35] Pearlman, D. A., D. A. Case, J. W. Caldwell, W. S. Ross, T. E. Cheatham, D. M. Ferguson, G. L. Seibel, U. C. Singh, P. K. Weiner, and P. A. Kollman. 1995. AMBER4.1. University of California, San Francisco

[36] Ross, W. S. 1995. CARNAL. University of California, San Francisco

[37] Saenger, W. 1983. Principle of Nucleic Acid Structure Springer-Verlag. New York.

[38] Sklenar, H., C. Etchebest, and R. Lavery. 1989. Describing protein structure: A general algorithm yielding complete helicoidal parameters and a unique overall axis. Proteins 6:46–60.

[39] Soumpasis, D. M., C. -S Tung, and A. E. Garcia. 1991. Rigorous description of DNA structures II. J. Biom. Struc. & Dyn. 8:867–888.

[40] Sprous, D., W. Zacharias, Z. A. Wood, and S. C. Harvey. 1995. Dehydrating agents sharply reduce curvature in DNAs containing A tracts. Nucl. Acid Res. 23:1816–1821.

[41] Stofer, E., and R. Lavery. 1993. Measuring the geometry of DNA grooves. Biopolymers 34:337–346.

[42] Swaminathan, S., Jr W. E. Harte, and D. L. Beveridge. 1991. Investigation of domain structure in proteins via molecular dynamics simulation: application to HIV-1 protease dimer. J. Amer. Chem. Soc. 113:2717–2721.

[43] Swaminathan, S., G. Ravishanker, D. L. Beveridge, R. Lavery, C. Etchebest, and H. Sklenar. 1990. Conformational and helicoidal analysis of the molecular dynamics of proteins. Proteins 8:179–193.

[44] Ulanovsky, L., M. Bodner, E. N. Trifonov, and M. Choder. 1986. Curved DNA: design, synthesis, and circularization. Proc. Natl. Acad. Sci. USA 83:862–866.
[45] Young, M. A., B. Jayaram, and D. L. Beveridge. 1997. Intrusion of counterions into the spine of hydration in the minor groove of B-DNA. J. Am. Chem. Soc. 119:59–69.
[46] Zhurkin, V. B. 1985. Sequence dependent bending and phasing of nucleosomes. J. Biomolec. Struct. Dyns. 2:785.

IONIC CHARGING FREE ENERGIES USING EWALD SUMMATION

TOM DARDEN*

Abstract. Recently, a number of groups have discovered that the use of Ewald summation leads to greatly improved stability in molecular dynamics simulations of nucleic acids, proteins and membrane bilayers. This presentation will discuss the effect of boundary conditions and treatment of long-range electrostatics on molecular dynamics simulations, as well as on the important problem of calculating free energy differences. Due to its simplicity, we focus on the problem of calculating ionic charging free energies. We review recent results that suggest Ewald summation gives appropriate values for this free energy, at least for the simple case of ion charging.

1. Introduction. The calculation of free energies of hydration is an important goal for molecular modelers. There are a large variety of methods available, ranging from rapid QSAR approaches to the free energy simulation approaches using explicit solvent. Currently, the free energy approaches are too expensive for routine use in the drug design process, but they do provide the most detailed understanding of interactions at the atomic level. Furthermore they alone are capable of providing a realistic description of the dynamics of the solvation process. Water both excites and damps motions in biomolecules in a way that has proven difficult to simulate without including explicit molecular solvent [1]. In addition, there are a growing number of experimental structures of proteins and protein-ligand complexes in which discrete water molecules are seen to play a key structural and energetic role [2]. These water molecules are not fixed, but rather exchange with bulk solvent, often on a time scale accessible to molecular dynamics simulations. The free energy approach is thus a natural choice for modeling these types of systems.

Two factors that limit the utility of free energy simulations to calculate solvation energies are errors in the force field representation of the system, and limitations in sampling enough of the relevant conformations of the system[3]. It is anticipated that both of these limitations will be alleviated with time. Force fields are continually being improved [4], while "*ab initio*" (Density Functional Theory) simulations of ions and small molecules in water, for periods of the order of 10 picoseconds, are already possible [5, 6]. Improvements in computer hardware and sampling algorithms [7] promise to relieve the conformational search problem for larger solutes. However, a third important factor which can limit the utility of free energy simulations is the choice of boundary conditions, together with the treatment of long-range electrostatics. As we will see, calculated free energies may vary depending on the boundary conditions used in a simulation, even if

*National Institute of Environmental Health Science Research, Triangle Park, NC 27709.

precisely correct atomic interactions can be calculated, and sampling issues fully overcome.

The issues involved are clearly illustrated by the simple case of calculating the free energy of charging an ion in water. The force field issues are straightforward; a standard water model is used, and the only remaining parameters are the Lennard-Jones attraction and repulsion parameters for interactions between the ion and water oxygen. In addition, sampling is not an issue, since converged values (to within a fraction of a kcal/mol) are routinely obtained. Despite this, the values obtained for this charging free energy have varied widely. The differences can be traced to the various treatments of boundary conditions and long-range electrostatics.

Although this chapter focuses on the use of periodic boundary conditions together with Ewald summation, we first discuss the more intuitive choice of free boundary or finite cluster calculations for molecular simulations. Recent results exploring the artifacts due to the solvent-vacuum boundary will be reviewed. After this we will introduce periodic boundary conditions and discuss the problem of long-range interaction in these boundary conditions, briefly deriving the Ewald summation method for handling Coulomb interactions. Next we review recent work characterizing the effect of the Ewald sum on molecular dynamics simulations in biomolecules. Finally we return to the problem of calculating ionic charging free energies. We introduce the problem by discussing the simpler case of continuum solvent in order to motivate the role of the self energy in explicit solvent simulations in finite spherical as well as periodic boundary conditions. Recent work on the subtle effects of long-range boundary conditions on the calculated energies is reviewed and it is suggested that at present the Ewald summation method gives the best approach to this problem.

2. Finite cluster simulations. As we will see below, the use of periodic boundary conditions in the context of Coulombic interactions leads to a host of subtle issues. It might be argued that a much simpler choice of boundary conditions for simulations involving explicit solvent is to surround the solute of interest with one or more layers of solvent, forming a finite cluster. The Coulomb interaction problem can be handled precisely by a simple sum over all atom pairs, and rapid approximations using the Fast Multipole Algorithm [8] make this approach feasible even for large systems. If desired, the dielectric effect of an infinite solvent surrounding the cluster can be modeled for example by reaction field [9] methods or the Langevin dipoles approach [10].

Unfortunately, this choice of boundary conditions can lead to a number of severe artifacts. These can all be traced to the non bulk-like behavior of the water molecules near the solvent-vacuum interface. The problem is best understood by examining the results of simulations of pure water using this choice of boundary conditions. While the behavior of water molecules near the center of such droplets is demonstrably bulk-like, as shown by Simonson's [11] calculation of a local dielectric constant, the density of water near the surface is anomolously low, as is its rate of rotational diffusion. The results of Essex and Jorgenson [12] show that these artifacts are not easily overcome, even for the simplest case of spherically symmetric clusters. The behavior of waters near the interface can also affect the results of free energy calculations. Wang and Hermans [9] studied the effect of ion position within a spherical water cluster on the calculated free energy of charging. For ions fixed at positions near the center of the sphere, the calculated free energies were nearly invariant to position. However, when the ion was positioned closer to the surface of the cluster, the calculated free energies changed markedly. Clearly, this problem would need to be addressed in calculations involving more complex solute shapes.

Despite the above concerns, if one is calculating the free energy of charging an ion, the choice of these boundary conditions, specifically a sufficiently large spherical cluster of solvent with the ion positioned at the center, would appear to be more suitable than the choice of periodic boundary conditions [13]. A priori, such a sphere should more closely approximate the ideal case of an isotropic, infinitely dilute ionic solution. However, as discussed below, even in this case the anomolous behavior of the waters near the surface can substantially affect the calculated energies, and this effect should not necessarily diminish with increasing system size.

3. Periodic boundary conditions and the Ewald sum. The above mentioned problems involving the interface between the system and the surrounding vacuum were well known to the pioneers of molecular simulation. Indeed, in the very first (Monte-Carlo) molecular simulation [14], periodic boundary conditions were chosen in order to better approximate bulk-like behavior. The systems studied initially, such as liquid argon, only involved short range interactions, and thus the implementation of periodic boundary conditions was straightforward. Atoms that crossed the surface of the (cubic) simulation cell were wrapped periodically, entering the opposite face. Interactions between atoms were computed under minimum image conditions; that is, for a cubic simulation cell of side L, the minimum image distance r'_{ij} between atom i at $\mathbf{r}_i = (x_i, y_i, z_i)$ and j at $\mathbf{r}_j = (x_j, y_j, z_j)$ is

$$r'_{ij} = |\mathbf{r}'_{ij}| = min_{\mathbf{n}}|r_i - r_j - \mathbf{n}L| \tag{1}$$

where $|\mathbf{r}| = (x^2 + y^2 + z^2)^{1/2}$ denotes the Cartesian length of the vector $\mathbf{r} = (x, y, z)$ and $\mathbf{n} = (n_1, n_2, n_3)$ is any triple of integers. Given an interaction potential $\phi_{ij}(\mathbf{r})$, where $\mathbf{r} = (x, y, z)$ is any point in Cartesian space, the minimum image interaction between atoms i and j is given by $\phi_{ij}(\mathbf{r}'_{ij})$. Often a further spherical cutoff was applied, so that interactions were only calculated if $r'_{ij} < R_C$ for some cutoff distance $R_C < L/2$.

Later, simulations of water and other molecular systems in which Coulombic interactions play an important role led to more complex considerations in the implementation of periodic boundary conditions. Whereas Lennard-Jones interactions are short-ranged, Coulombic interactions are long-ranged. This can be traced to the fact that the three dimensional sum

$$\sum_{\mathbf{n}\neq\mathbf{0}} \frac{1}{|\mathbf{n}|^p} \tag{2}$$

is finite for $p > 3$, but infinite for $p \leq 3$. Thus, if $\mathbf{r} = (x, y, z)$ is a point in Cartesian space with Cartesian length $r = |\mathbf{r}| = (x^2+y^2+z^2)^{1/2}$, and $\phi_{ij}(\mathbf{r})$ an interaction potential, ϕ_{ij} is considered short ranged if, for some $\delta > 0$, $r^{3+\delta} \cdot \phi_{ij}(\mathbf{r})$ converges to zero as $r \to \infty$ and is long-ranged otherwise. For N atoms at positions $\mathbf{r}_i, i = 1, \ldots, N$ in a cubic simulation cell of length L, the potential energy of the system under periodic boundary conditions is given by the sum

$$U = \frac{1}{2} \sum_{\mathbf{n}}{}' \sum_{i,j=1}^{N} \phi_{ij}(\mathbf{r}_i - \mathbf{r}_j - \mathbf{n}L) \tag{3}$$

where $\mathbf{n}$ denotes the integer triple (n_1, n_2, n_3) and the prime on the outer sum means that the self terms with $i = j$ are not computed when $\mathbf{n} = (0, 0, 0)$. If ϕ_{ij} is short ranged, then referring to equation 2 we see that the infinite sum involved in the potential energy converges absolutely. Furthermore, for sufficiently large simulation cells, the potential can be safely approximated using a spherical cutoff as above, that is

$$U = \frac{1}{2} \sum_{\mathbf{n}}{}' \sum_{i,j=1}^{N} \phi_{ij}(\mathbf{r}_i - \mathbf{r}_j - \mathbf{n}L) \approx \sum_{i<j} \phi_{ij}(\mathbf{r}_{ij}^{'})\chi(r_{ij}^{'} < R_C) \tag{4}$$

where χ is the indicator function. On the other hand, if ϕ_{ij} is long-ranged, as is true for Coulombic and dipolar interactions, the potential energy will either diverge or converge conditionally, meaning that the result depends on the order of summation. In addition, even for large simulation cells it is not safe to approximate using a spherical cutoff.

It thus might seem hopeless to meaningfully calculate electrostatic interactions under periodic boundary conditions, but nature provides a model in the form of ionic crystals which are effectively infinite periodic structures. In this case $\phi_{ij}(\mathbf{r})$ is given by $q_i q_j/|\mathbf{r}_i - \mathbf{r}_j|$ where q_i and q_j are the atomic charges of the ions i and j. For example in the sodium chloride crystal each sodium atom interacts electrostatically with all of its own periodic images except itself, as well as all periodic images of the chloride atom in the same unit cell. The resulting lattice energy can be experimentally measured, providing a check on the calculation.

Among the methods that have been developed to treat the problem of Coulombic lattice sums, the Ewald summation has been the most successful. To arrive at the Ewald sum, imagine a point charge q positioned at the center of the cubic cell and consider the problem of calculating the electrostatic potential at some other point $\mathbf{r}$ in the cell due to that point charge and all its periodic images. Manifestly, this potential is infinite, and so we must first neutralize the charge by filling the cell with a uniform neutralizing plasma which has density $-q/L^3$ and thus total charge $-q$, and which is also periodically replicated. Now imagine a spherically symmetric gaussian charge density surrounding the point charge, also having total charge $-q$, and also periodically replicated. The electric field at any point in the cell due to the point charge and its gaussian counterion density may be easily calculated from Gauss' law. The integral of this field gives a potential $q\ \mathrm{erfc}(\beta r)/r$ at $\mathbf{r}$, where β is the width of the gaussian. The potential due to the periodic images of the point charge plus gaussian counterion density are obtained similarly, and the total summed to give the Ewald direct sum. Since we added the gaussian counterion density, we need to cancel this effect by adding a gaussian co-ion density having total charge q and the same width β, which is then periodically replicated. The potential due to the smooth periodic source given by the uniform charge density $-q/L^3$ and the gaussian co-ion density can be obtained by solving Poisson's equation in periodic boundary conditions, resulting in the Ewald reciprocal sum. Finally, since the potential is only specified up to an arbitrary constant, we choose this by insisting that the average potential over the simulation cell be zero. The electrostatic potential at $\mathbf{r} \neq \mathbf{0}$ is then $q\ \psi(\mathbf{r})$ where the Ewald potential $\psi(\mathbf{r})$ is given by

$$\psi(\mathbf{r}) = \sum_{\mathbf{n}} \frac{\mathrm{erfc}(|\mathbf{r}+\mathbf{n}|)}{|\mathbf{r}+\mathbf{n}|} + \frac{1}{\pi L} \sum_{\mathbf{m}\neq 0} \frac{\exp(-\pi^2 m^2/\beta^2)}{m^2} \exp(2\pi \mathbf{m}\cdot\mathbf{r}/L) - \frac{\pi}{\beta^2 L^3}$$

(5)

The self-term or Wigner potential [15] is given by $q\ \zeta$ where $\zeta = \lim_{r\to\infty} (\psi(r) - 1/r)$, and is the electrostatic potential at the origin due to the nontrivial periodic images of the point charge together with the neutralizing plasma and its images. For cubic unit cells $\zeta \approx -2.8373/L$. Finally, the potential energy of a unit cell consisting of N point charges q_i at $\mathbf{r}_i$ together with their compensating uniform plasmas (which have no effect if the sum of the charges is zero) is given by

$$U_{ew} = \sum_{i<j} q_i q_j \psi(r'_{ij}) + \frac{\zeta}{2} \sum_{i=1}^{N} q_i^2 \tag{6}$$

In the above derivation we have, after applying the uniform neutralizing plasma, replaced a conditionally convergent sum by a pair of rapidly absolutely convergent sums. Clearly, something has been thrown away in the process. This issue was finally resolved rigorously by DeLeeuw, Perram and Smith [15] who considered the effect of summation order explicitly. In particular they discussed the potential energy of a cubic unit cell with N point charges as above, at the center of a finite spherical array of periodic replicas of itself, taking the limit as the sphere expanded to infinity. They found the limiting potential energy was given by $U_{ew} + 2\pi M^2/L^3$ where $\mathbf{M} = q_1 r_1 + \ldots + q_N r_N$ is the dipole moment of the central cell. They then discussed the effect of immersing the spherical array in a dielectric continuum, arriving at a reaction field term depending also on the dipole moment of the central cell. When the dielectric constant was infinite, corresponding to conducting boundary conditions, this reaction field term precisely cancelled the above dipole term, giving back the original Ewald sum. Most workers prefer to use the Ewald sum without the dipolar correction term, probably because including the extra term destroys the periodicity of the potential. However, recently Boresch and Steinhauser [16] have demonstrated the advantages of using the extra term with a finite dielectric constant, at least for calculation of the dielectric constant of a simulated liquid.

4. Molecular dynamics simulations using Ewald sums. Although the use of Coulombic lattice sums is clearly appropriate for the treatment of ionic crystals, its use in liquid state molecular simulations has been questioned, due to the resulting amplification of instantaneous dipolar fluctuations [17] within the simulation cell. A reasonable physically motivated alternative is the reaction field approach, in which explicit Coulombic interactions are truncated spherically at a cutoff radius while interactions of more distant charges are modeled as the response of a dielectric continuum to the total dipole moment of the charges in the cutoff sphere centered on the charge of interest. This approach has the added benefit of restoring spherical isotropy to the interaction potential, in place of the artificial cubic symmetry of the Ewald pair potential. As stated, the reaction field approach is only appropriate for systems where the cutoff sphere is net-neutral. However it can be generalized to charged systems [18].

Although the use of lattice sum techniques in liquid simulations was questioned a priori, results of such simulations using Ewald sum techniques have been remarkably consistent with those using reaction field methods [19]. Thus, at least for these systems, the concerns about inappropriate amplification of dipolar fluctuations have been shown to be unfounded.

In the biomolecular simulation community, the Ewald sum has not been used until recently, probably due mainly to its significant computational cost. The Ewald sum as usually implemented is an order N^2 algorithm in the number of point charges, while the straightforward cutoff techniques are of order N. Furthermore, applying a cutoff to a long-range interaction, while theoretically inappropriate, was not widely felt to be a major problem, compared to limitations in the force fields used. Finally, due to the highly anisotropic nature of these simulation cells, consisting of a large biomolecule, often highly charged, surrounded by a layer of water to fill out the simulation cell, the earlier experiences with Ewald sums in the liquid state community would not necessarily be relevant to these systems.

However, more recently, at about the same time algorithmic advances made Ewald summation possible in large systems [20], a number of groups discovered severe problems with the use of cutoffs in biomolecular simulations. A particularly clear example is given by Auffinger and Beveridge [21]. They simulated a system consisting of an equal number of sodium and chloride ions in a periodic box of TIP3P water, using various choices for a molecule based cutoff. Regardless of the cutoff used, they found a large peak in the sodium-sodium and chloride-chloride radial distribution function at the cutoff boundary. Evidently the system was able to lower its energy by eliminating unfavorable interactions through the use of a cutoff. Earlier, Hagler and coworkers [22] reported similar findings with respect to charged sidechains in simulations of a solvated protein using cutoffs. A number of groups experienced disastrous results when applying cutoff techniques in simulations of DNA, whereas the use of Ewald methods led to stable simulations [23]. More recently, some groups have reported stable simulations of DNA [24] using a more sophisticated atom based force switching cutoff with a large cutoff radius [25]. Interestingly, these more sophisticated cutoff approaches appear to be related to the family of reaction field methods [26]. However, all of the available cutoff methods were shown to produce highly artifactual behavior in simulations of a water vapor interface, and to distort at least some aspects of membrane simulations [27]. Interestingly, in these latter cases, it is the cutoff methods which lead to long-range amplification of structural disturbances at the boundary, destroying bulk-like fluid behavior in the interior of the systems, whereas the use of Ewald sums clearly damps out the surface structure, preserving an isotropic liquid interior.

Although Ewald summation has been shown to lead to stable simulation in a variety of biomolecular simulations, it is a priori possible that it does so by suppressing fluctuations, "freezing in" certain modes of the system due to "overemphasis" of the periodicity. For example, a macromolecule with a large net dipole might experience inhibited rotation in the cell due to interactions with its periodic images. Smith and Pettitt [28, 29] have demonstrated that these artifacts are of minor importance, at least in high dielectric solvents near room temperature. More complex dynamic artifacts due to Ewald summation may yet emerge. However, the exciting finding by Cheatham and Kollman [30] that DNA oligonucleotides simulated using the PME [31] approximation to Ewald sums converge rapidly to a stable B-like structure independent of the starting structure shows that Ewald summation does not inhibit conformational search. Thus, recent experience indicates that the use of periodic boundary conditions, together with Ewald summation to treat the long-range interactions, appears to be the method of choice for carrying out molecular dynamics simulations of solvated biomolecules.

5. Free energy of ionic charging. Although artifacts in structural or dynamic properties of the simulated system associated with the use of Ewald summation appear to be minimal, at least for high dielectric solvents, the use of Ewald sums in free energy calculations might still be questioned. Figueirido *et al.* [32] and Luty and van Gunsteren [33] have reported significant finite system effects on interaction energies involving pairs of charges. These effects decay only slowly with larger simulation cells. As yet there is little experience to indicate whether these artifacts will seriously affect calculated free energy changes in biomolecules, and if they can be simply corrected.

Due to its simplicity, it is instructive to focus on the calculation of the free energy of charging an ion in a cubic simulation cell under periodic boundary conditions. This problem has been studied very thoroughly in a series of papers by Hummer *et al.* [34, 35, 36] and we will mainly review their findings as well as responses of others to them.

It is helpful to begin by discussing a simpler continuum model of charging an ion. We imagine a spherical cavity with internal dielectric constant equal to one and radius R immersed in an infinite dielectric continuum having dielectric constant ϵ. A point charge at the center of the cavity is slowly charged from charge-state q_0 to q_1. At any point $\mathbf{r} \neq 0$ the electrostatic potential $\phi(q;\mathbf{r})$, where the argument q denotes the dependence on the charge state q, gives the work of bringing a unit test charge from infinity to $\mathbf{r}$ and includes contributions from the polarized dielectric medium as well as the direct Coulomb interaction with the point charge at the center of the cavity. Note that the potential ϕ, which in general includes an arbitrary constant C, is defined uniquely by insisting that $\phi(q;\mathbf{r}) \to 0$ as $r \to \infty$. Thus the energetic cost, due to the polarization of the medium, in bringing the test charge in from infinity is given by $\phi(q;\mathbf{r}) - q/r$, and the work done in charging the ion from q_0 to q_1 is

$$W = \int_{q_0}^{q_1} \lim_{r\to 0}(\phi(q;\mathbf{r}) - q/r)dq \tag{7}$$

By Gauss' law and the spherical symmetry it is easy to see that for $r > R$, $\phi(q;\mathbf{r}) = q/(\epsilon r)$, while for $0 < r < R$, $\phi(q;\mathbf{r}) = q/r - q/R + q/(\epsilon R)$, and thus the work done on the medium in charging the ion is given by $W = -1/2(1 - 1/\epsilon)(q_1^2 - q_0^2)/R$, which is the familiar Born expression.

If the infinite dielectric continuum is replaced by a large sphere of molecular solvent with the ion at the origin, the instantaneous (configuration dependent) value of $\phi(q;\mathbf{r})$ is given by q/r plus the potential contributions $q_i/|\mathbf{r}_i - \mathbf{r}|$ of the other atoms in the system, and thus, averaging over the molecular configurations at each charge state of the central ion, the work done by the molecular solvent in charging the ion is given by

$$(8) \quad W = \int_{q_0}^{q_1} < \lim_{r \to 0}(\phi(q;\mathbf{r}) - q/r) >_q dq = \int_{q_0}^{q_1} < \sum_{i=1}^{N} q_i/r_i >_q dq$$

where the sum is over the atoms of the solvent and the $< \ldots >_q$ denotes the average over configurations at charge state q.

This result can be compared to the above Born expression. To the extent the bath of water molecules behaves like a linear dielectric, we can expect similar values for the charging free energy. Of course, in this case the hard sphere cavity of the ion is replaced by a van der Waals potential. Furthermore, the molecular nature of the solvent, in particular that of the solvent layer closest to the ion, whose behavior is insensitive to simulation artifacts due to boundary conditions or the treatment of long-range electrostatics, manifests itself in deviations from the linear dielectric response assumed by the Born model [37, 38], particularly when comparing positive versus negative ionic charge states [34]. Thus given sufficiently accurate interaction potentials, molecular simulations should give more informative and accurate values for charging free energies.

However, in the case of spherical water clusters the artifactual behavior of the solvent molecules near the surface can bias the results of charging free energy calculations. This problem was discussed by Hummer *et al.* [35] in the context of calculating the electrostatic potential of a neutral Lennard-Jones particle in a bath of solvent, or more specifically $< \lim_{r\to 0}(\phi(q;\mathbf{r}) - q/r) >_q$ at charge state $q = 0$. Clearly this value is zero for the simple continuum model. The values reported for explicit solvent simulations have varied. Hummer *et al.* [34] report a positive value, whereas Aqvist [37] reports a negative value. Hummer *et al.* [35] explain the discrepancies by differences in the methods used to sum the electrostatic potential over the water bath They recommend calculating the average electrostatic potential by integrating q/r against the radial distribution function of the hydrogen and oxygen atoms. This seems physically correct, since the radial distribution is an experimental observable. Hummer *et al.* demonstrate that the electrostatic potential of an uncharged Lennard-Jones particle in a periodic box of solvent, simulated with Ewald conditions and calculated using atomic radial distribution functions, agrees with the average Ewald electrostatic potential. The latter is the configurational average of the sum of $q_i\psi(\mathbf{r}_i)$ over the atoms of the solvent, where ψ is the Ewald pair potential discussed above and $\mathbf{r}_i$ the displacement of atom i with respect to the Lennard-Jones particle. Similar conclusions were reached by Ashbaugh and Wood [39].

Hummer *et al.* [35] also simulated the same Lennard-Jones particle at the center of water clusters of various sizes, using Coulombic interactions with no cutoff, and calculated the electrostatic potential at the particle as a function of radial distance along the radial distribution function of the solvent atoms. They showed that the accumulated potential reached a plateau within the cluster, oscillating about a value which agreed with the (positive) average potential given by the Ewald sum. However, as the radial distance approached the radius of the sphere the non bulk-like behavior of the surface waters caused a large artifactual adjustment to the calculated potential. Due to the long-ranged nature of Coulombic interactions, this adjustment is not expected to be alleviated by increasing the cluster size. Clearly, free energies calculated in cluster simulations should not include interactions between solute atoms and waters near the surface, and should be accumulated using the radial distribution function approach of Hummer *et al.*

Before discussing the calculation of charging free energies using explicit solvent under periodic boundary conditions, it is again helpful to look at a simpler continuum model. We imagine a model, where the spherical cavity of radius R containing the point charge is at the center of a cubic box of side L with $R < L/2$. The rest of the cube is filled with a dielectric continuum having dielectric constant ϵ. The whole system is then periodically replicated. At a given charge state q, the potential $\phi(q;\mathbf{r})$ for points $\mathbf{r}$ in the cube can be obtained by solving Poisson's equation separately in the two dielectric domains, with the source given by the point charge q together with a uniform neutralizing plasma, while enforcing periodic boundary conditions and appropriately matching the two solutions at the cavity boundary. Hummer *et al.* [36] used cubic harmonic polynomials [40] to approximate the potential $\phi(q;\mathbf{r})$. Again the solution includes an arbitrary constant C. This was set by insisting that the average of $\phi(q;\mathbf{r})$ over the simulation cell be zero, as with the Ewald potential ψ. Taking the limit of an infinite dielectric constant and assuming R is small compared to $L/2$, they found that $\lim_{r\to 0}(\phi(q;\mathbf{r}) - q/r) \approx -q/R + 2\pi q R^2/L^3$, and the work done on the medium in charging the ion could be approximated by $W = -1/2(q_1^2 - q_0^2)(1/R - 2\pi q R^2/L^3)$. Thus, at least within the dielectric continuum theory, for a high dielectric medium the effects of periodic boundary conditions should be minor.

A number of groups, beginning with Straatsma and Berendsen [41], have attempted to calculate free energies of ionic charging using explicit solvent and periodic boundary conditions. The simulations of Straatsma and Berendsen employed a finite cutoff of the ion-solvent and solvent-solvent interactions. They report inconsistent results when varying these cutoff parameters, with or without the use of a Born correction to correct for finite system effects. These inconsistencies were clarified later by Wood [42], who developed a correction term for the solvent-solvent cutoff, showing that it led to consistent system-size independent results. He also compared his results with those of Aqvist [13], who also obtained consistent system-size independent results using finite cluster calculations, which however differed from Wood's by roughly 5 kcals/mol for the sodium ion. Wood suggested these differences could be traced to Aqvist's inclusion of interactions between the ion and non bulk-like waters near the cluster boundary. Hummer *et al.* [34] calculated free energies of charging for a number of ions, using the parameters of Straatsma and Berendsen [41], and the Ewald method. They emphasize the importance of the self-energy term ζ in correcting for finite system effects. Using this self-energy term they report consistent system-size independent results which however differed by roughly 20 kcals/mol for sodium from those of Wood and Aqvist. They also report simulations using a generalized reaction field approach which agree with their Ewald results. Later, Ashbaugh and Wood [39] were able to explain the differences between their results and the Ewald results in terms of the molecule-based versus atom-based accumulation of potential at the ion position. That is, using the same radial distribution based integration of the potential as suggested by Hummer *et al* [35], they obtain results much closer to the Ewald results. They attribute the remaining small discrepancies to unphysical structuring in the solvent radial distributions near the cutoff. Thus, at this time it seems that the ionic charging free energies obtained by Ewald summation are correct for the interaction potentials used, although definitive studies of cluster simulations have yet to be done. Questions associated with the use of periodic boundary conditions and Ewald summation remain, however. As pointed out by Bogusz *et al.* [43], the size consistency of the Ewald results is somewhat mysterious, in that identical results hold for very small system sizes where the solvent cannot be expected to act as a high dielectric liquid. They also point out significant size dependent pressure artifacts which could bias simulations. In correcting for these artifacts however, they destroy the size consistency of the charging free energy results, although they obtain the same result in the limit of large systems, or more rapidly with a Born-type correction.

In summary, recent results point to a possible resolution of the question of how to correctly calculate the free energy of ionic charging using molecular dynamics simulations with explicit solvent. This question is important, since as noted in the introduction, the methodological issues associated with boundary conditions remain even if more sophisticated force fields or even *ab initio* interaction potentials are employed in free energy calculations. Hopefully the progress made on the simple ionic systems will help us understand how to correctly calculate free energy differences in more complex systems.

REFERENCES

[1] P. E. SMITH AND B. M. PETTITT, *Modeling solvent in biomolecular systems*, J. Phys. Chem., **98**:9700–9711, 1994.

[2] J. E. LADBURY, *Just add water: The effect of water on the specificity of protein-ligand binding sites and its potential application to drug design*, Chemistry and Biology, **3**:973–982, 1996.

[3] P. KOLLMAN, *Free energy calculations: Applications to chemical and biochemical phenomena*, Chem. Rev., **93**:2395–2417, 1993.

[4] P. Kollman, *Advances and continuing challenges in achieving realistic and predictive simulations of the properties of organic and biological molecules*, Acc. Chem. Res., **29**:461–469, 1996.

[5] M. Parrinello, *From silicon to rna: The coming of age of ab initio molecular dynamics*, Solid State Commun., **102**:107–120, 1997.

[6] M. E. Tuckerman, P. J. Ungar, T. von Rosenvinge, and M. L. Klein, *Ab initio molecular dynamics simulations*, J. Phys. Chem., **100**:12878–12887, 1996.

[7] B. J. Berne and J. E. Straub, *Novel methods of sampling phase space in the simulation of biological systems*, Curr. Opin. Str. Bio., **7**:181–189, 1997.

[8] L. Greengard and V. Rokhlin, *A fast algorithm for particle simultations*, J. Comp. Phys., **73**:325–348, 1987.

[9] Lu Wang and Jan Hermans, *Reaction field molecular dynamics simulation with Friedman's image charge method*, J. Phys. Chem., **99**:12001–12007, 1995.

[10] Arieh Warshel and Michael Levitt, *Theroretical studies of enzymatic reaction: Dielectric, electrostatic and steric stabilization of the carbonium ion in the reaction of lysozyme*, J. Mol. Biol., **103**:227–249, 1976.

[11] Thomas Simonson, *Accurate calculation of the dielectric constant of water from simulations of a microscopic droplet in vacuum*, Chem. Phys. Lett., **250**:450–454, 1996.

[12] Jonathan W. Essex and William L. Jorgensen, *An empirical boundary potential for water droplet simulations*, J Comp. Chem., **16**:951–972, 1995.

[13] J. Aqvist, *Ion-water interaction potentials derived from free energy perturbation simulations*, J. Phys. Chem., **94**:8021–8024, 1990.

[14] N. Metropolis, A. Rosenbluth, M. Rosenbluth, and E. Teller, *Equation of state calculations by fast computing machine*, J. Chem. Phys., **21**:1087–1092, 1953.

[15] S. W. DeLeeuw, J. W. Perram, and E. R. Smith, *Simulation of electrostatic systems in periodic boundary conditions I: Lattice sums and dielectric constants*, Proc. R. Soc. Lond., **A373**:27–56, 1980.

[16] S. Boresch and O. Steinhauser, *Presumed versus real artifacts of the ewald summation technique: The importance of dielectric boundary conditions*, Ber. Bunseges. Phys. Chem., **101**:1019–1029, 1997.

[17] J. P. Valleau and S. G. Whittington, *A guide to Monte Carlo for statistical mechanics: 1. Highways*, In B. J. Berne, editor, *Statistical Mechanics, Part A: Equilibrium Techniques*, **volume 5**, New York, NY, 1977, Plenum.

[18] G. Hummer, D. M. Soumpasis, and M. Neumann, *Computer simulation of aqueous Na-Cl electrolyte*, J. Phys. Condens. Matt., **23A**: A141–A144, 1994.

[19] S. W. DeLeeuw, J. W. Perram, and E. R. Smith, *Computer simulation of the static dielectric constant of systems with permanent dipole moments*, Ann. Rev. Phys. Chem., **37**:245–270, 1986.

[20] A. Toukmaji and J. A. Board, *Ewald sum techniques in perspective: A survey*, Comp. Phys. Comm., **95**:78–92, 1996.

[21] Pascal Auffinger and David L. Beveridge, *A simple test for evaluating the truncation effects in simulations of systems involving charged groups*, Chem. Phys. Lett., **234**:413–415, 1995.

[22] David H. Kitson, Franc Avbelj, John Moult, Dzung T.Nguyen, John E. Mertz, D. Hatzi, and Arnold T. Hagler, *On achieving better than 1 Ångstrom accuracy in a simulation of a large protein: Streptomyces griseus protease A*, Proc. Nat. Acad. Sci., **90**:8920–8924, 1993.

[23] S. Louise-May, P. Auffinger, and E. Westhof, *Calculations of nucleic acid conformations*, Curr. Opin. Str. Biol., **6**:289–298, 1996.

[24] A. D. MacKerrell, *Influence of magnesium ions on duplex dna structural, dynamic, and solvation properties*, J. Phys. Chem. B, **101**:646–650, 1997.

[25] P. J. Steinbach and B. R. Brooks, *New spherical cutoff methods for long-range forces in macromolecular simulation*, J. Comp. Chem., **15**:667–683, 1994.

[26] Lalith Perera, Ulrich Essmann, and Max L. Berkowitz, *Effect of the treat-*

ment of long-range forces on the dynamics of ions in aqueous solutions, J. Chem. Phys., **102**:450–456, 1995.

[27] S. E. Feller, R. W. Pastor, A. Rojnuckarin, S. Bogusz, and B. R. Brooks, *Effect of electrostatic force truncation on interfacial and transport properties of water*, J. Phys. Chem., **100**:17011–17020, 1996.

[28] P. E. Smith and B. M. Pettitt, *Ewald artifacts in liquid state molecular dynamics simulations*, J. Chem. Phys., **105**:4289–4293, 1996.

[29] P. E. Smith and B. M. Pettitt, *On the presence of rotational ewald artifacts in the equilibrium and dynamical properties of a zwitterionic tetrapeptide in aqueous solution*, J. Phys. Chem. B, **101**:3886–3890, 1997.

[30] T. E. Cheatham III and P. A. Kollman, *Observation of the a-dna to b-dna transition during unrestrained molecular dynamics in aqueous solution*, J .Mol. Bio., **1996**:434–444, 259.

[31] Ulrich Essmann, Lalith Perera, Max L. Berkowitz, Tom Darden, Hsing Lee, and Lee G. Pedersen, *A smooth particle mesh Ewald method*, J. Chem. Phys., **103**:8577–8593, 1995.

[32] F. Figuerido, G. S. Del Buono, and R. M. Levy, *On finite-size effects in computer simulations using the Ewald potential*, J. Chem. Phys., **103**:6133, 1995.

[33] B. A. Luty and W. F. van Gunsteren, *Calculating electrostatic interactions using the particle-particle particle-mesh method with nonperiodic long-range interactions*, J. Phys. Chem., **100**:2581–2587, 1996.

[34] G. Hummer, L. R. Pratt, and A. E. Garcia, *On the free energy of ionic hydration*, J. Phys. Chem., **100**:1206–1215, 1996.

[35] G. Hummer, L. R. Pratt, A. E. Garcia, B. J. Berne, and S. W. Rick, *Electrostatic potentials and free energies of solvation of polar and charged molecules*, J. Phys. Chem. B, **101**:3017–3020, 1997.

[36] G. Hummer, L. R. Pratt, and A. E. Garcia, *Ion sizes and finite-size corrections for ionic-solvation free energies*, J. Chem. Phys., **107**:9275–9277, 1997.

[37] J. Aqvist and T. Hansson, *On the validity of electrostatic linear response in polar solvents*, J. Phys. Chem., **100**:9512–9521, 1996.

[38] S. W. Rick and B. J. Berne, *The aqueous solvation of water: A comparison of continuum methods with molecular dynamics*, J. Am. Chem. Soc., **116**:3949–3954, 1994.

[39] H. Ashbaugh and R. Wood, *Effects of long-range electrostatic potential truncation on the free energy of ionic hydration*, J. Chem. Phys., **106**:8135–8139, 1997.

[40] D. Adams and G. Dubey, *Taming the Ewald sum in the computer simulation of charged systems*, J. Comp. Phys., **72**:156–176, 1987.

[41] T. P. Straatsma and H. J. C. Berendsen, *Free energy of ionic hydration: Analysis of a thermodynamic integration technique to evaluate free energy differences by molecular dynamics simulations*, J. Chem. Phys., **89**:5876–5886, 1988.

[42] R. H. Wood, *Continuum electrostatics in a computational universe with finite cutoff radii and periodic boundary conditions: Correction to computed free energies of ionic solvation*, J. Chem. Phys., **103**:6177–6187, 1995.

[43] S. Bogusz, T. Cheatham III, and B. Brooks, *Removal of pressure and free energy artifacts in charged periodic systems via net charge corrections to the ewald potential*, J. Chem. Phys., 1998, in press.

GENETIC FUNCTION APPROXIMATION: EVOLUTIONARY CONSTRUCTION OF NOVEL, INTERPRETABLE, NONLINEAR MODELS OF EXPERIMENTAL DATA

DAVID ROGERS*

Abstract. Genetic Function Approximation (GFA) is a technique for generating statistical models of data using the process of evolution. Replacing regression analysis with the GFA algorithm allows the construction of models competitive with, or superior to, standard techniques and makes available additional information not provided by other techniques. Unlike most other analysis algorithms, GFA provides the user with multiple models; the populations of models are created by evolving random initial models using a genetic algorithm. GFA can build models using not only linear polynomials but can also be used to generated nonlinear models containing splines. These spline-based models are often novel when compared to models from standard methods, and are easily-interpretable by a domain expert. In this paper, two examples of the application of GFA are discussed. The first is an example of quantitative structure-property relationship (QSPR) modeling, in which structure changes in molecular are correlated with a physical property of interest. The second is a formulation modeling example, in which the concentrations of the components of a mixture are correlated with some physical property of the product obtained from the mixture.

Key words. Genetic algorithms, statistical modeling, experimental design, regression methods, property prediction, quantitative structure-property relationships, quantitative structure-activity relationships, formulations.

> "If your experiment needs statistics,
> you ought to have done a better experiment"
>
> – *Ernest Rutherford*

1. Introduction. Notwithstanding the negative appraisal of the value of statistics by the Nobel prize winning physicist Ernest Rutherford, statistical modeling has proven to be an important and powerful tool for discovery and understanding of underlying relationships in experimental data set. This paper describes one such modeling method, called the Genetic Function Approximation (GFA) algorithm, and illustrates its strength in nonlinear modeling against two real-world data sets.

The Genetic Function Approximation (GFA) algorithm is a technique for generating statistical models of data using the process of evolution [1,2,3], derived from earlier work on evolutionary spline modeling [4,5]. This method stands in contrast to techniques such as stepwise regression [6] partial-least squares regression [7,8], or neural-net modeling [9], which deterministically construct a single functional model of a data set from a given set of first principles and assumptions. Unlike these methods, GFA

*Currently at Molecular Simulations Incorporated, 9685 Scranton Road, San Diego, CA 92121-3752. Net address: drogers@msi.com

uses a nondeterministic process analogous to evolution to guide the development of a population of many statistical models. Further, the method is naturally amenable to the construction of nonlinear models of data: by allowing the models to have nonlinear terms, such as higher-order polynomials or spline-based terms, the population will develop novel, easily-interpreted, and statistically-reasonable nonlinear models.

The current popularity of neural-network models derives in part from their status as an easily-applied method for generating nonlinear models of data. Unfortunately, issues such as lack of interpretability, overfitting, difficulty of selection of the appropriate network size and structure, and distance from the extensive work on statistical modeling limit their utility. Work on spline-based modeling such as Friedman's Multivariable Adaptive Regression Splines (MARS) [10] suggests one alternative, but often such algorithms are limited to data sets of moderate size.

This chapter will promote GFA as a possible alternate to both neural-networks and spline-modeling algorithms. After a brief description of GFA, the remainder of the chapter will develop in depth two real-world examples of the use of GFA for nonlinear modeling. The first example is from the field of quantitative structure-property relationship (QSPR) modeling; in this domain, the goal is to build a model relating physico-chemical parameters of molecules to a molecular property. The second example is from the formulations area; in this domain, the goal is to build a model relating the relative concentrations of components of a mixture to a physical property of the product of the mixture.

2. Description of the genetic function approximation algorithm. Many techniques develop a regression model by incremental addition or deletion of basis functions to a single model. The primary idea of GFA is to keep a *population* of models, and use the genetic algorithm to recombine among these models. By selecting "parent" models which are representing the data set better than the average model, and creating a "child" model from parts of each parent, the child model has an increased probability of being as good as or better than the parents at representing the data.

The basic form of the models is shown in Figure 1. The model is assumed to be a linear sum of basis functions times coefficients $\{a_k\}$. At the start of the program, the basis functions are chosen randomly. The model coefficients $\{a_k\}$ are determined using least-squares regression. In this way, a collection of many models is created.

Each model in the population is represented as a series of basis functions, which are the terms of the model. Each model is represented as a linear string of basis functions, as shown in Figure 2. The basis functions, denoted by greek letters, can be any function of the independent variables contained in X; examples are $x_1, \sin(x_2 - x_1 + 1)$ and $(x_4 - .4)(x_5 - .1)$. The output of the model, denoted $F(X)$, is an estimator of the value of the

$$F(X) = a_0 + \sum_{k=1}^{M} a_k \, \phi_k(X)$$

FIG. 1. *The basic form of the models developed by GFA.*

dependent variable given the values of the independent variables contained in X. For quantitative structure-property relationship (QSPR) studies, the dependent variable is a physical property of a compound or mixture; for quantitative structure-activity relationship (QSAR) studies, the dependent variable is some biological activity of a compound.

$$\begin{array}{l} F_1 : \{\phi_1\, \phi_2\, \phi_3\, \phi_4\, \phi_5\, \phi_6\, \phi_7\, \phi_8\, \phi_9\, \phi_{10}\, \phi_{11}\, \phi_{12}\, \phi_{13}\, \phi_{14}\} \\ F_2 : \{\delta_1\, \delta_2\, \delta_3\, \delta_4\, \delta_5\, \delta_6\, \delta_7\, \delta_8\, \delta_9\, \delta_{10}\, \delta_{11}\} \\ \vdots \qquad\qquad\qquad \vdots \\ F_k : \{\sigma_1\, \sigma_2\, \sigma_3\, \sigma_4\, \sigma_5\, \sigma_6\, \sigma_7\, \sigma_8\, \sigma_9\, \sigma_{10}\, \sigma_{11}\, \sigma_{12}\} \end{array}$$

FIG. 2. *Representation of the population of models.*

Once the basis functions of a model are chosen, and the coefficients calculated, the model is scored using a variant of Friedman's "lack of fit" (LOF) measure [10], which is a penalized least-squares measure for goodness of fit; this measure takes into account factors such as the n, the number of data samples; LSE, the least-squares error; c, the number of nonconstant basis functions; p, the total number of parameters in the model; and d, a user-settable parameter which, by default, has the value 1.0. The LOF measure is shown in Figure 3.

$$\text{LOF} = \frac{LSE}{\left(1 - \frac{c+(d \times p)}{n}\right)^2}$$

FIG. 3. *Friedman's lack-of-fit (LOF) measure.*

Use of this error measure (rather than the more common least-squares error (LSE) or correlation-coefficient (r)) greatly reduces the tendency towards overfitting. "Good" models are those which predict the dependent variable with both the least error and the least complexity.

Once the population of models is constructed, we repeatedly perform the *genetic crossover* operation:

- Two good models are probabilistically selected as "parents". The likelihood of being chosen is inversely proportional to a model's LOF score.
- Each parent is randomly "cut" into two sections, and a new model is created using a piece from each parent. The crossover operation is shown in Figure 4.

$\underline{\phi_1\ \phi_2\ \phi_3\ \phi_4\ \phi_5\ \phi_6}\ \phi_7\ \phi_8\ \phi_9\ \phi_{10}\ \phi_{11}\ \phi_{12}\ \phi_{13}\ \phi_{14}$	First parent
$\delta_1\ \delta_2\ \delta_3\ \delta_4\ \delta_5\ \underline{\delta_6\ \delta_7\ \delta_8\ \delta_9\ \delta_{10}\ \delta_{11}}$	Second parent
$\downarrow \qquad \downarrow \qquad \downarrow$	
$\underline{\phi_1\ \phi_2\ \phi_3\ \phi_4\ \phi_5\ \phi_6\ \delta_6\ \delta_7\ \delta_8\ \delta_9\ \delta_{10}\ \delta_{11}}$	New model

FIG. 4. *The crossover operation.*

- (Optional *mutation* operators may alter the newly-created model.)
- The model with the worst LOF score is replaced by this new model.

This process ends when the average LOF score of the models in the population changes less than some user-determined value e over some predetermined number of generations. Unlike most neural-network techniques, there is little risk of overfitting if the evolution is allowed to run for a lengthy period. This is because the complexity of the constructed model is determined *explicitly* through the LOF function rather than *implicitly* by the length of training.

The GFA process is a search of the space of possible models for models which optimize the value of the LOF score. In particular, it can discover models with combinations of features that work well together, but which may not be easily discovered individually.

(The GFA algorithm is described in more detail in [1].)

2.1. Nonlinear modeling with splines. One of the strengths of GFA is its ability to discover potential *nonlinear* relationships in data set and expose them in an easily-interpreted form to the user. While GFA can use standard quadratic, cubic, or other power terms in its basis functions to reflect some nonlinear effects, it is often preferable to capture nonlinearities directly using *spline-based terms.*

GFA uses a class of splines called *truncated power splines*, which are denoted using angle brackets: $\mathbf{f}(\mathbf{X}) =< \mathbf{X} - \mathbf{a} >$, where "$\mathbf{X}$" is the variable and "$\mathbf{a}$" is a constant called the *knot* of the spline. The value of the function is 0.0 if $\mathbf{X} <= \mathbf{a}$ and $(\mathbf{X} - \mathbf{a})$ if $\mathbf{X} > \mathbf{a}$. A plot of this function is shown in Figure 5. Similarly, the spline function $\mathbf{f}(\mathbf{X}) =< \mathbf{a} - \mathbf{X} >$ is defined as 0.0 if $\mathbf{X} >= \mathbf{a}$ and $(\mathbf{a} - \mathbf{X})$ if $\mathbf{X} < \mathbf{a}$, as shown in Figure 6.

An advantage of this formulation of splines is that the location of the nonlinearity is made explicit: it is the value "$\mathbf{a}$" in the descriptor

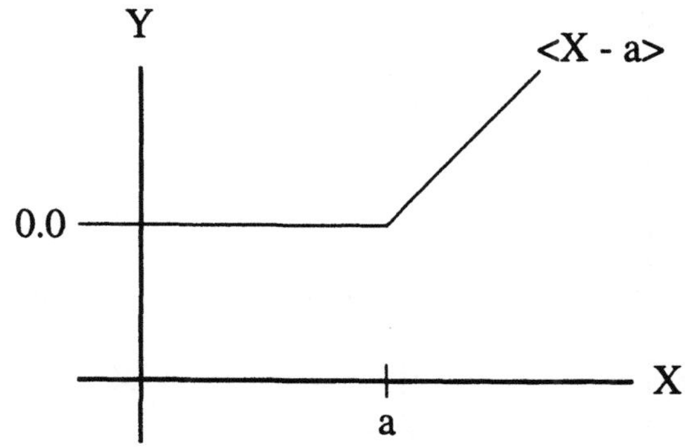

FIG. 5. *Plot of spline function* $< \mathbf{X} - \mathbf{a} >$.

"**X**". In effect, the spline term is partitioning the samples in the data set depending on the value of a given descriptor. Thus, it can represent relationships between descriptors and the response that are only linear in a limited region of the descriptor values. This is a common situation when modeling experimental data, where a theoretically-expected linear relationship often breaks down for extreme values of a given descriptor.

An important feature of splines in modeling is that they are *interpretable*: they make the location and effect of the nonlinearity explicit to the user. This is in contrast to neural-network techniques, which can obscure the location and effect of nonlinearities between the independent and dependent variables.

3. Example 1. The Log*P* data set. The octanol-water partition coefficient (Log$P$) is a useful property of organic compounds in that it often reflects transport-related behavior directly related to bioactivity. It is also useful in estimating solubility-related physical properties of commercial interest. The utility of this measure, combined with the difficulty and expense of obtaining it through direct measurement, has created a demand for computational methods for estimating it. The most widely-used methods are based upon *group contributions*, in which tables of substituents and their associated contribution values are used to estimate Log$P$ for a set of compounds with a similar core structure.

Quantitative structure-property relationship (QSPR) techniques are methods which use statistical modeling to correlate changes in molecular structure with physical properties. Each row of a data table is associated with a given molecular structure; the columns contain experimental or computational descriptions of each molecule. Statistical modeling is used to correlate the molecular properties with a property of interest.

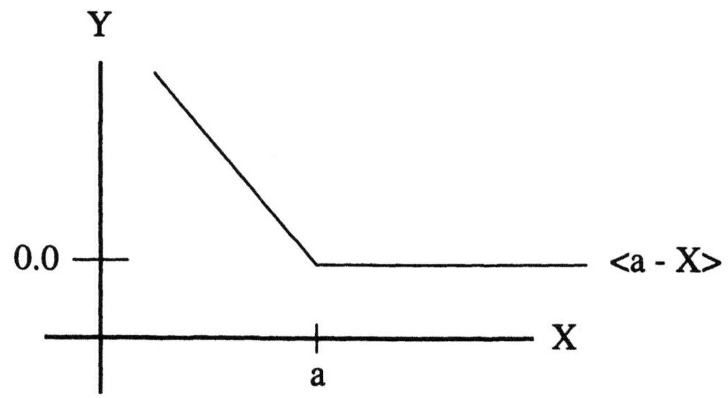

FIG. 6. *Plot of spline function* $< \mathbf{a} - \mathbf{X} >$.

In the past, statistical modeling using general molecular descriptors have been used to estimate Log*P*, but only within specific compound classes. More recently, Moschner and Cece [11] report success in using QSPR techniques to build a broadly-applicable model of Log*P*. Such a model would prove useful in cases where group contribution methods perform poorly, as with the prediction of the Log*P* of polyethoxylated nonionic surfactants.

The Moschner and Cece model was built for a total of 191 compounds and a table of 50 descriptors. The final model retained 12 descriptors. These descriptors of the model are shown in Figure 7. The "fraction" column is denoted by [brackets], and is the relative contribution of that descriptor to the model.

Using the provided data set of the 12 descriptors, the authors' model was reproduced by fitting the terms with a PLS fit using mean centering, scaling, and 6 components. This model is shown in Figure 8. As with the descriptor list, the numbers in [brackets] to the right of each term of the model are the fractions of model output that a given term is responsible for.

3.1. GFA analysis. GFA analysis was conducted using the full 191 sample data set containing 12 variables. Linear polynomial terms and linear spline terms were allowed in the models. The original population of models contained 100 randomly-constructed models, and it was evolved for 10,000 crossover steps. The best model (as rated by LOF) is shown in Figure 9. The terms of the model are ordered by the fraction of response they are responsible for.

Descriptor	Description	Fraction
BASICITY	Most negative charge on a heteroatom	0.193
CHG_C_3	Total charge on sp^3 carbon atoms	0.121
C_AR	Number of aromatic carbon atoms	0.110
LOG_MW	Log of the molecular weight	0.095
DIPOLE	Dipole moment	0.093
VOLUME	Molecular volume	0.081
AMINO_AC	Amino acid flag: 1 for amino acids	0.080
N_AR	Number of aromatic nitrogen atoms	0.043
CHG_C_AR	Total charge on aromatic carbons	0.054
CHG_O_3	Total charge on sp^3 oxygens	0.054
N_3	Number of sp^3 nitrogen atoms	0.039
HYDROCAR	Hydrocarbon flag	0.037

FIG. 7. *Descriptors used in LogP modeling.*

3.2. Interpretation of the terms of the GFA model. Most notable are the first two terms, two splines based upon the descriptor CHG_O_3, which is the total charge on sp^3 oxygens. These two terms together account for about a 45% fraction of the response. (Interestingly, this same variable was responsible for less than a 5.5% fraction of the response in the linear PLS model.)

The spline terms are categorizing the samples into three groups based upon their value of CHG_O_3: more negative than -0.400 (about 22 samples), between -0.400 and -0.304 (about 72 samples), and more positive than -0.304 (about 97 samples). The effective coefficient of CHG_O_3 for the first group is $(-6.5810 + 3.9917) = -2.5893$; for the second group, 3.9917; for the third, 0.0. A graph of the relative effect of CHG_O_3 on the response is shown in Figure 10.

For the samples in the third group, the CHG_O_3 terms contribute nothing to Log$P$. Starting at value -0.304, then getting more negative, there is a sharp positive effect on Log$P$, peaking at -0.400 with a maximum correction value of +0.383. There is a more gradual fall-off of the correction value as the values get more negative, down to a correction of 0.0 at a value of -1.458. Extreme values of CHG_O_3 cause a negative correction of Log$P$. (Only three compounds in this set have values of CHG_O_3 more negative than -1.458; interestingly, two of them are in the class of polyethoxylated nonionic surfactants.)

The interpretation of nonlinearities can take either of two forms: either the physical process as reflected in a descriptor is truly nonlinear (in this case, that there would be a physical reason why CHG_O_3 would have this effect on Log$P$), or the descriptor is being used to categorize the data (in this case, the interpretation is that some subclass of the samples are being effectively grouped by a descriptor value). The choice can only be made

LOGP = −1.919522

+	5.562730	*	BASICITY	[0.193]
+	−2.983449	*	CHG_C_3	[0.121]
+	0.170498	*	C_AR	[0.110]
+	2.410511	*	LOG_MW	[0.094]
+	−0.149251	*	DIPOLE	[0.092]
+	0.006775	*	VOLUME	[0.081]
+	−2.642864	*	AMINO_AC	[0.079]
+	1.594764	*	CHG_C_AR	[0.054]
+	0.687514	*	CHG_O_3	[0.053]
+	−0.896965	*	N_AR	[0.042]
+	−0.863016	*	N_3	[0.038]
+	−0.609086	*	HYDROCAR	[0.037]

N: 191	LSE: 0.376
LOF: 0.492	r^2: 0.864
r^2_{adj}: 0.855	F: 94.017
SSE: 71.793	SSR: 455.042

FIG. 8. *The 6-component PLS model for LogP. The numbers in [brackets] are the loadings of each term; in effect, these are the relative importance of each term in the model. The statistics are: the number of samples (N); least-squares error (LSE); Friedman's lack-of-fit (LOF); Spearman's correlation coefficient squared (r^2) and the adjusted correlation coefficient squared (r^2_{adj}); F-test: (F); sum of squared errors (SSE); sum of squared residuals (SSR).*

by inspection by a scientist, which is why the interpretability of a model is critical.

The descriptor BASICITY also uses two spline terms, and accounts for about 22% of the response. A graph of the effect of values of BASICITY on Log*P* is shown in Figure 11.

In this graph, increasingly negative BASICITY exerts a negative correction on Log*P*. From its most positive values to −0.327, it has a steady linear relationship. (This group contains about 74 compounds). From −0.327 to −0.394, no further correction is made. (This group contains about 64 compounds). More negative than −0.394 leads to a sharper negative correction. (This group contains about 53 compounds).

(While we graph separate terms of the model as an aid to interpretation, it should be noted that all the terms of the model are selected by the genetic algorithm to work well as a group; it may be that the given nonlinear relationships are only appropriate because information in other variables is performing other corrections on Log*P*.)

Again, whether this nonlinear behavior is from an effective categorization of the samples or is a reflection of nonlinearities in the physical relationship between BASICITY and Log*P* is a question that is best answered by the interpreting scientist.

$$
\begin{array}{llcll}
\multicolumn{5}{l}{\text{LOGP}_{\text{GFA-1}} = -1.2930} \\
+ & -6.5810 & * & < -0.400 - \text{CHG\_O\_3} > & [0.278] \\
+ & 3.9917 & * & < -0.304 - \text{CHG\_O\_3} > & [0.176] \\
+ & -9.9505 & * & < -0.394 - \text{BASICITY} > & [0.161] \\
+ & 0.0204 & * & \text{VOLUME} & [0.160] \\
+ & -3.2326 & * & \text{AMINO\_AC} & [0.063] \\
+ & 5.7830 & * & < \text{BASICITY} - -0.327 > & [0.061] \\
+ & 2.4032 & * & < 0.132 - \text{CHG\_C\_3} > & [0.053] \\
+ & 0.1040 & * & \text{C\_AR} & [0.044]
\end{array}
$$

N: 191	LSE: 0.258
LOF: 0.330	r^2: 0.906
r^2_{adj}: 0.902	F: 220.323
SSE: 49.308	SSR: 477.526

FIG. 9. *The top-rated GFA model for LogP.*

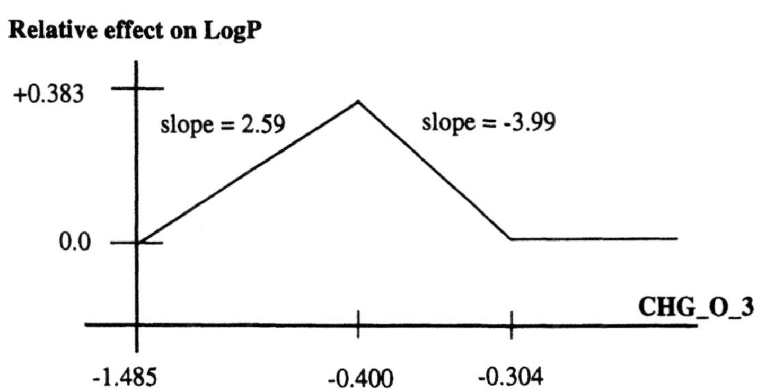

FIG. 10. *Plot of* $f = -6.5810 * < -0.400 - CHG\_O\_3 > +3.9917 * < -0.304 - CHG\_O\_3 >$.

3.3. Interpretation of the statistics of the GFA model. Two statistic types are available in judging the quality of the GFA model. The first group of statistics is statistics of the model as applied to the training set. These are measures of how well the model represents the information in the training set. The second group is statistics of the model applied against the test set. The statistics for the GFA model against the test set, and the results of applying the model against the samples, are shown in Table 1.

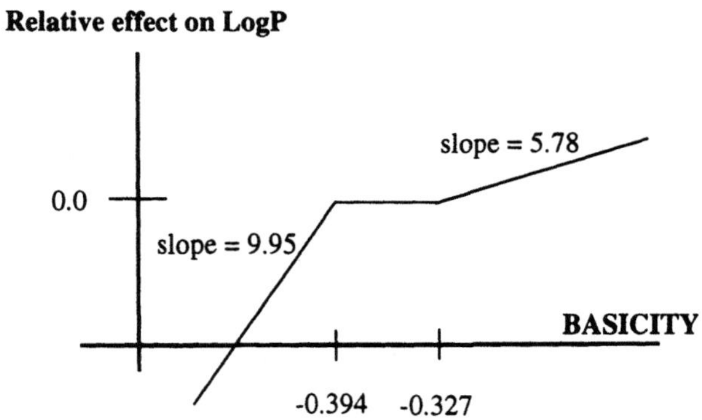

FIG. 11. *Plot of* $f = -9.9505 * < -0.394 - BASICITY > +5.7830 * < BASICITY - -0.327 >$.

TABLE 1
The predictions and residuals for PLS and GFA models vs. the test set.

Test#	Log(P)	Pred_{PLS}	Res_{PLS}	Pred_{GFA}	Res_{GFA}
1	−0.620	−0.011	−0.011	−0.277	0.342
2	−1.720	0.079	1.799	−0.669	1.050
3	0.460	0.201	−0.259	0.533	0.073
4	3.590	3.292	−0.298	2.971	−0.618
5	3.180	2.466	−0.714	2.495	−0.684
6	0.460	0.506	0.046	0.681	0.221
7	1.880	1.792	−0.088	2.427	0.547
8	4.110	4.104	−0.005	4.178	0.068
9	−0.920	1.153	2.073	0.890	1.810

LSE_{PLS}: 0.954 $\quad$ LSE_{GFA}: 0.634
r^2_{PLS}: 0.834 $\quad$ r^2_{GFA}: 0.900

A number of interesting points can be made about the top-rated GFA model as compared to the PLS model.

- The statistics on the training set show the GFA model to be equivalent or superior to the model derived using PLS.
- The GFA model gave better predictions on the 9 test compounds as measured either by least-square error (LSE) or r^2.
- The GFA model uses 8 terms and a constant, as versus 12 terms and a constant for the PLS model. Further, it uses only 6 of the 12 variables available in the data set. The model is simpler in the sense

that it explains Log$P$ using a more compact set of descriptors and fewer terms. (It is more difficult to estimate the degrees of freedom used by each model, as this measure is not easily defined for either spline-based terms or PLS components.)

- The variable DIPOLE is not used; this leaves VOLUME as the only conformationally-dependent variable in the model. Thus, the GFA model may be more applicable in cases where conformational modeling is difficult, expensive, or leads to large variations in the values of DIPOLE and hence renders any model using DIPOLE prone to error.

3.4. GFA and PLS models against anionic surfactants. The training set contains a subset of samples of special importance: a set of surfactants that are difficult to estimate using standard group contribution methods for estimating Log$P$. The predictions of both the PLS model and the GFA model against the anionic surfactants in the training set are broken out in Table 2.

TABLE 2
PLS vs. GFA against the anionic surfactants in the training data.

Sample	Obs Log$P$	PLS Pred	PLS Resid	GFA Pred	GFA Resid
167	−0.45	1.04	−1.49	−0.48	0.02
168	−0.35	0.15	−0.50	−0.39	0.04
169	−1.38	−0.20	−1.18	−0.47	−0.90
170	−1.38	0.27	−1.65	−0.34	−1.03

In all classes, the GFA model performed as well or better than the PLS model. In the difficult case of anionic surfactants, the GFA model performed better than the PLS model, though there were still appreciable residuals in 2 of the 4 compounds. One possible reason for the better performance of the GFA model may be due to the lack of DIPOLE in the model. As stated in the original article, more polarized and charge-separated compounds such as 167-170 can have large differences in the value of DIPOLE depending on the chosen conformation. The GFA model, by using information independent of the DIPOLE descriptor (and thus avoiding the conformation issue), may be able to offer better predictions for this class.

3.5. Discussion of QSPR results. This paper presents work on using GFA to re-analyze a data set previously analyzed using partial least-squares (PLS) regression. By using GFA with nonlinear terms, a nonlinear model of Log$P$ was constructed which was compact, used fewer descriptors, avoided the troublesome DIPOLE descriptor, had better statistics on the training and test sets, and suggested unique interpretations and insights into the data that were not seen in the PLS analysis.

This is not a critique of PLS as a general analysis technique; for certain kinds of data, it is an excellent method for capturing information spread over many variables when few training samples are available. Indeed, recent work by myself and Dr. W.J. Dunn III demonstrates a combination of GFA and PLS called Genetic Partial Least Squares (G/PLS) [2] that combines the ability of GFA to find predictive combinations of variables with PLS's smooth-fitting abilities. The reason for the weakness of PLS in this case was that important information in the data set was nonlinear, and such information is not easily discovered using PLS or other linear modeling techniques. Application of nonlinear modeling methods such as neural-networks is a possibility, but the price paid is a lack of interpretability of the final model, which then must be taken on faith.

The GFA model studied above was not the only possible model; in fact, GFA generated many model with similar statistics. The top 8 nonlinear GFA models of Log$P$, along with some running commentary, are given in Appendix A. The existence of *multiple models* for a given data set is not surprising; for most experimental data, the solution is *underdetermined*, hence many statistically-equivalent models (hypotheses) are possible.

While not discussed here, these multiple models are not merely left-overs to be discarded; instead, they are critical if the user wishes to *predict* the value of new samples, or *design experiments* to enrich the data set further [12]. For example, if a given test sample leads to widely-varying predictions among the different statistically-equivalent models (that is, different hypotheses predict different things), then that prediction is not to be trusted. However, in the case of experimental design, the situation is reversed: such samples make excellent experiments, and by adding them preferentially to the training set, one guides the discovery process to rapidly differentiate between physically-valid and merely fortuitous hypotheses. The payoff is both more-predictive models and a greater understanding of the relationship between the parameters at hand and the underlying physical system.

This study is preliminary, and could be easily extended. For example, a variety of other molecular descriptors could be calculated to augment the given Log$P$ data set. GFA or other variable-selection techniques could then be applied to discover whether any of these new descriptors are bringing unique information to the process.

4. Example 2. The flare brilliance data set. The flare brilliance data set is a formulations data set which attempts to relate the brightness of flares with the concentrations of 4 components.

A *formulations* study is a modeling task in which the independent variables contain concentration information about components in a mixture, and the dependent variables contains information about a property of the product developed from the mixture. For example, a plastic formulation might use two substances: a polymer monomer base and a polymerization accelerant. The property of interest might be the hardness of the resulting plastic. Each row of the data table contains information from a different mixture. The columns might contain three independent variables: the concentration of the polymer monomer base, the concentration of the polymerization accelerant, and a variables which is the multiplicative product of the two concentrations; this last variable can reflect interaction effects between the former two components. Once the table is constructed, standard statistical modeling techniques can be used to postulate a relationship between the independent variables and the hardness of the plastic.

This example will use the example of McLean and Anderson [13] who published an investigation of the illumination of flares. The experimental data for the study is contained in Table 1. The concentrations of the components in each experiment were derived using standard experimental design methods.

TABLE 3
The flare brilliance data set.

Sample	Magnesium	Sodium Nitrate	Strontium Nitrate	Binder	Illumination
	Mg	**$NaNO_3$**	**$SrNO_3$**	**Binder**	
1	.4	.1000	.4700	.030	75
2	.4	.1000	.4200	.080	180
3	.6	.1000	.2700	.030	195
4	.6	.1000	.2200	.080	300
5	.4	.4700	.1000	.030	145
6	.4	.4200	.1000	.080	230
7	.6	.2700	.1000	.030	220
8	.6	.2200	.1000	.080	350
9	.5	.1000	.3450	.055	220
10	.5	.3450	.1000	.055	260
11	.4	.2725	.2725	.055	190
12	.6	.1725	.1725	.055	310
13	.5	.2350	.2350	.030	260
14	.5	.2100	.2100	.080	410
15	.5	.2225	.2225	.055	425

This table was augmented before analysis by adding columns for the products of the concentrations of each of the 4 components. The final table contained 10 independent variables and 1 independent variable, which was a measurement of the brightness of the flare with the given composition.

In the standard analysis, a model for illumination was derived from a 15-point design to fit a 10-term Scheffé quadratic model, as shown in Figure 12.

The study continued by eliminating the cross-terms involving the binder as "nonsignificant": thus, **(Mg * Binder)**, **($NaNO_3$ * Binder)**,

$$
\begin{array}{llcl}
\multicolumn{4}{l}{\mathbf{Illumination}_{\text{10-term}} =} \\
 & -1551 & * & \mathbf{Mg} \\
+ & -2348 & * & \mathbf{NaNO_3} \\
+ & -2423 & * & \mathbf{SrNO_3} \\
+ & 18183 & * & \mathbf{Binder} \\
+ & 8320 & * & (\mathbf{Mg} * \mathbf{NaNO_3}) \\
+ & 8096 & * & (\mathbf{Mg} * \mathbf{SrNO_3}) \\
+ & -10870 & * & (\mathbf{Mg} * \mathbf{Binder}) \\
+ & 3239 & * & (\mathbf{NaNO_3} * \mathbf{SrNO_3}) \\
+ & -21265 & * & (\mathbf{NaNO_3} * \mathbf{Binder}) \\
+ & -21393 & * & (\mathbf{SrNO_3} * \mathbf{Binder})
\end{array}
$$

$$r^2 = 0.86 \; ; \quad r^2_{\text{adj}} = 0.607$$

FIG. 12. *The 10-term Sheffé model for illumination using all 10 independentvariables.*

and (**$SrNO_3$ * Binder**) were deleted to give the reduced model as shown in Figure 13. According to the original authors, "the r^2_{adj} values are not as high as is typically desired".

$$
\begin{array}{llcl}
\multicolumn{4}{l}{\mathbf{Illumination}_{\text{7-term}} =} \\
+ & -929 & * & \mathbf{Mg} \\
+ & -2205 & * & \mathbf{NaNO_3} \\
+ & -2287 & * & \mathbf{SrNO_3} \\
+ & 3666 & * & \mathbf{Binder} \\
+ & 6519 & * & (\mathbf{Mg} * \mathbf{NaNO_3}) \\
+ & 6297 & * & (\mathbf{Mg} * \mathbf{SrNO_3}) \\
+ & 3288 & * & (\mathbf{NaNO_3} * \mathbf{SrNO_3})
\end{array}
$$

$$r^2 = 0.823 \; ; \quad r^2_{\text{adj}} = 0.690$$

FIG. 13. *The reduced 7-term model for illumination.*

In order to formalize this intuitive estimation, leave-one-out cross-validation was performed.[1] In this test, each sample is removed from the data set in turn, and regression used to construct a model from the remaining data samples. The left-out sample is predicted with the newly-generated model. This process results in a score called the *cross-validated* r^2 (XV-r^2 or q^2). An intuitive meaning can be attached to this score: it is

[1]It should be noted that cross-validation is not typically used against data sets generated through experimental design: because each point is carefully chosen to cover its region of design space, leaving it out forces an extrapolation from the remaining points, resulting in scores that can be unjustly poor. The "true" predictivity of the model might be higher.

the percentage of variance in the dependent variable that is explained by the model.

When performed against the 10-term model, the cross-validation test results in a negative score, which means the model is nonpredictive. (That is, one would be better off always guessing the mean value of the dependent variables rather than using the model.) For the 7-term model, the cross-validated r^2 was 0.166. That is, the model explained only about 16% of the variance of the illumination. This confirms the intuition of the original authors: neither model shows acceptable predictive ability.

4.1. Linear GFA modeling of illumination data. Genetic Function Approximation was applied to this data set, creating models that contained only linear terms from the data set. (The next section will explore nonlinear modeling of the data set.) The evolution started with a population of 100 randomly-generated models which were evolved for 10,000 generations. The top 3 models (as rated by Friedman's LOF score) are shown in Figure 14.

Illumination$_{\text{GFA-L1}}$ =	**Illumination**$_{\text{GFA-L2}}$ =	**Illumination**$_{\text{GFA-L3}}$ =
255 * **Mg**	638 * (**Mg** * **NaNO$_3$**)	8600 * (**Mg** * **Binder**)
+ 4527 * (**Mg** * **Binder**)	+ 6501 * (**Mg** * **Binder**)	
r^2 = 0.498	r^2 = 0.489	r^2 = 0.438
r^2_{adj} = 0.459	r^2_{adj} = 0.431	r^2_{adj} = 0.259
XV-r^2 = 0.353	XV-r^2 = 0.316	XV-r^2 = 0.129

FIG. 14. *Top 3 models for illumination generated by GFA.*

The models are certainly different from the standard models. Their predictive values are still weak (XV-r^2 from 0.129 to 0.353), but two of the three models showing superior predictiveness to the standard 7-term model.

Of more interest, the models are *smaller, simpler to interpret* and *use different terms* from the 7- and 10-term models. The length of the models are determined during the evolution by the LOF measure, which balances the least-squares error of the model (how well it has learned the data) with the complexity of the model. In this case, only a few terms appeared to be justifiable.

The interpretability of the models is a reflection of their form and smaller size. In these models, it is only the concentration of magnesium (Mg) and its interaction with the binder (Mg * Binder) that are used. Such simple models are more likely to provoke the scientist to a simple hypothesis about the underlying physical system, and to suggest simple experiments that can test the hypothesis.

Finally, the GFA models use different terms from the 7- and 10-term models. Because of their small size, many terms must be discarded. But the remaining terms may also be different: in all 3 top models, the interaction variable (Mg * Binder) was used; this term was discarded as nonsignificant in the standard study of the data set. Offering different models to the scientist is more likely to allow them to use their scientific knowledge to identify factors that may have remained hidden in the standard analysis.

4.2. Nonlinear GFA modeling of illumination data. As shown in the previous section, nonlinear modeling with GFA can expose nonlinear effects that can both improve model predictivity and offer unique possibilities for scientific interpretation. In this case, we repeated the analysis from the previous section, but in this case allowed both linear terms and linear spline terms. The top-rated model is shown in Figure 15.

$$\text{Illumination}_{\text{GFA-N1}} = \; = -767$$

$$\begin{array}{lrcl} + & 1802 & * & \mathbf{Mg} \\ + & 3567 & * & \mathbf{Binder} \\ + & 409 & * & (\mathbf{Mg} * \mathbf{NaNO_3}) \\ + & -12715 & * & < 0.047- (\mathbf{NaNO_3} * \mathbf{SrNO_3}) > \end{array}$$

$$r^2 = 0.952; \qquad r^2_{\text{adj}} = 0.933$$
$$\text{XV}-r^2 = 0.90$$

FIG. 15. *The top-rated nonlinear GFA model for illumination.*

Of most interest is the great increase in the cross-validated r^2. By capturing a nonlinear effect, we are now predictively explaining 90% of the variance. Because the LOF measure weights linear and spline terms differently, not all terms are used nonlinearly, unlike other nonlinear modeling methods such as neural-networks. A rule of thumb is that a spline term "costs" as much to include as two linear terms. This creates a pressure to use splines only when there is a large predictive payback, and assists in keeping models simple and interpretable.

The model contains one nonlinear term: an interaction term involving sodium nitrate ($NaNO_3$) and strontium nitrate ($SrNO_3$). This spline term is equal to 0.0 when the product ($NaNO_3$ * $SrNO_3$) is greater than or equal to 0.047, and positive as the product gets smaller. Given the large negative coefficient of the spline term in the model, it suggests that illumination is reduced when the joint concentration of the two salts falls below the given level. While it does not directly suggest a physical model for the importance of this interaction (do the salts co-crystallize? is the mixing process of the salts failing?...), it is effective at pointing the scientist at a key area that deserves further study. Such insights into the physical system are often more important than any given predictive model, which may or may not be used further.

The top 8 nonlinear GFA models of illumination, along with some running commentary, are given in Appendix B.

4.3. Validation of GFA process. However, some statistical caution is in order before the models suggested by GFA should be accepted. The cross-validation process we used early validated the model, but not the variable selection and spline construction steps of GFA. Thus, perhaps the cross-validation score is fortuitous, and is only due to lucky variable selection or spline construction.

This hypothesis can be testing in two ways: by doing a *full cross-validation*, and by performing a *randomization* test.

Full cross-validation is a procedure to validate, not a model, but a process for constructing models. Each sample is left out in turn. Then, the analysis procedure (in this case, GFA) is performed using the remaining samples to generate a best model. This model is used to predict the value of the left-out sample. When performed using nonlinear GFA against the illumination data set, the full cross-validated r^2 is 0.76. Thus, the nonlinear GFA process is constructing models which predictively explains over 76% of the variance.

A randomization test is a test to answer the question: what is the likelihood that the model came from a random chance? In this process, the r^2 of the model resulting from the application of a method to the data set is calculated. Then, the dependent variable is randomized, and the process used to generate a model of the randomized data set. The r^2 of the model from this process is compared to the r^2 of the model from the nonrandomized data set. By repeating this randomization a number of times, we can increase our confidence that the model is not from random chance. For example, Figure 16 shows a histogram of 99 randomized runs, and the r^2's of the resulting models. Given that the r^2 of the nonrandomized model was superior to all 99 randomized models, we can say that the nonlinear GFA model is not the product of chance at the 99% confidence level.

5. Conclusions. This chapter described a method for statistical model construction called Genetic Function Approximation or GFA. It described the GFA algorithm, then demonstrated its utility in developing novel, interpretable models of experimental data by showing results from applying it to two previously-studied real-world data sets.

In both cases, GFA discovered models that would have been overlooked by modeling with established methods. Indeed, given the large differences between the GFA models and the models presented in the original works, a strong case can be made that, at the minimum, a method such as GFA should be used to augment standard modeling methods. By offering the scientist disparate models of data from a physical system, the opportunity for the scientist to use their domain-based knowledge and insight is increased.

Further, in both cases, the use of splines during the GFA process offered novel, interpretable models that outperformed the standard linear

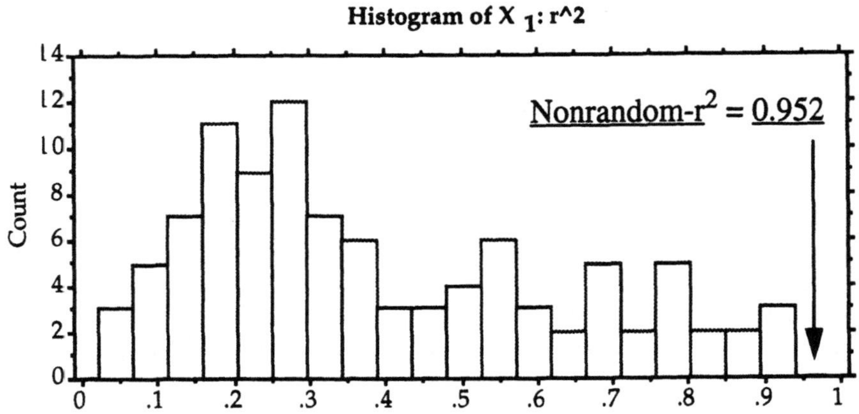

FIG. 16. *Results of randomization test of nonlinear GFA against the illumination data set.*

models of the data set. By making the location and nature of the nonlinearities explicit, the user is quickly focused on important relationships that exist in the training data.

Finally, the generation of multiple models of a given data set seems more appropriate that generating a single, "take-it-or-leave-it" model. This is especially true when the experimental data is *underdetermined*, that is, does not contain enough information to differentiate among alternate hypotheses of the system. By providing these alternatives models, the user has two new opportunities: if the models agree on their prediction for a given sample, that prediction is likelier safer (since all competing hypotheses agree); if the model differ in their predictions, accepting any one prediction is risky, though the sample is an excellent candidate for experimental design, that is, a sample for which much would be learned if the experiment is performed. New work, called *Evolutionary Statistics* [12], exploits this property of multiple models to integrate run-time prediction validation and experimental design to maximize learning.

In conclusion, GFA offers a simple, validated method for generating novel and interpretable nonlinear models of experimental data. Rather than directly competing with other nonlinear modeling techniques, it offers unique features that may make it the method of choice for data sets in which interpretability and model simplicity are of paramount importance.

Acknowledgements. David Rogers wishes to thank Drs. Moschner and Cece for supplying the data set used in the QSPR study, and for their efforts in supplying the molecular structures in an appropriate format. Aileen Alvarado-Swaisgood provided much time, advice, and effort

$LOGP_{GFA\text{-}1} = -1.2930$

+	−6.5810	*	< −0.400− CHG_O_3>	[0.278]
+	3.9917	*	< −0.304− CHG_O_3>	[0.176]
+	−9.9505	*	< −0.394− BASICITY>	[0.161]
+	0.0204	*	VOLUME	[0.160]
+	−3.2326	*	AMINO_AC	[0.063]
+	5.7830	*	<BASICITY − −0.327 >	[0.061]
+	2.4032	*	< 0.132− CHG_C_3>	[0.053]
+	0.1040	*	C_AR	[0.044]

N: 191	LSE: 0.258
LOF: 0.330	r^2: 0.906
r^2_{adj}: 0.902	F: 220.323
SSE: 49.308	SSR: 477.526

FIG. 17. *Model 1 out of 8.*

$LOGP_{GFA\text{-}2} = -1.338189$

+	−9.6699	*	< −0.393− CHG_O_3>	[0.331]
+	7.2086	*	< −0.303− CHG_O_3>	[0.256]
+	0.0190	*	VOLUME	[0.120]
+	6.0027	*	BASICITY	[0.109]
+	−3.3958	*	AMINO_AC	[0.053]
+	−3.3754	*	< −0.395− BASICITY>	[0.044]
+	−1.5838	*	CHG_C_3	[0.033]
+	1.3435	*	LOG_MW	[0.027]
+	0.0645	*	<C_AR>	[0.022]

N: 191	LSE: 0.264
LOF: 0.338	r^2: 0.904
r^2_{adj}: 0.899	F: 189.810
SSE: 50.473	SSR: 476.362

FIG. 18. *Model 2 out of 8.*

in preparing the data and molecules for analysis, and supplied the original suggestion that I do this study. Matt Hahn provided me the time to work on this study (thanks Matt!) away from my busy duties. Doug Brockman patiently waited while I took long trips developing this work. Marvin Waldman lent a kind scientific ear to my ideas in their formative stages. And Mike Doyle deserves much credit for being a strong and constant voice in the development of data analysis tools such as GFA to formulations and QSPR tasks.

$LOGP_{GFA\text{-}3} = -1.3546$

+	−13.7674	*	< −0.393− CHG_O_3>	[0.354]
+	10.4952	*	< −0.303− CHG_O_3>	[0.280]
+	0.0252	*	VOLUME	[0.119]
+	8.0826	*	BASICITY	[0.110]
+	0.1511	*	<C_AR>	[0.038]
+	−3.6089	*	< 0.0− CHG_C_AR>	[0.038]
+	−3.1913	*	AMINO_AC	[0.037]
+	−0.9524	*	CHG_C_AR	[0.012]
+	−0.4743	*	CHG_C_3	[0.007]

N: 191	LSE: 0.264
LOF: 0.337	r^2: 0.904
r^2_{adj}: 0.900	F: 190.189
SSE: 50.381	SSR: 476.453

FIG. 19. *Model 3 out of 8.*

$LOGP_{GFA\text{-}4} = 0.7007$

+	−9.6553	*	< −0.399− CHG_O_3>	[0.333]
+	6.8272	*	< −0.304− CHG_O_3>	[0.245]
+	0.0214	*	VOLUME	[0.136]
+	5.1049	*	BASICITY	[0.094]
+	−4.5415	*	< −0.395− BASICITY>	[0.060]
+	−3.3005	*	AMINO_AC	[0.052]
+	2.4707	*	< −0.052− CHG_C_3>	[0.038]
+	0.1004	*	<C_AR>	[0.034]
+	0.1668	*	HYDROCAR	[0.005]

N: 191	LSE: 0.267
LOF: 0.345	r^2: 0.903
r^2_{adj}: 0.898	F: 187.465
SSE: 51.043	SSR: 475.792

FIG. 20. *Model 4 out of 8.*

APPENDIX

A. The top 8 nonlinear GFA models for Log*P*. Model 1 of 8 has been previously discussed in the text. It uses 6 out of the 12 possible variables. It shares with all other top 8 models the use of the two spline terms on variable CHG_O_3, though the knot positions are slightly adjusted for some of the models. All top 8 models share a linear term for each of VOLUME and AMINO_AC. Finally, all top 8 models use BASICITY, though some use it linearly, and others use a spline of BASICITY.

$\text{LOGP}_{\text{GFA-5}} = 0.8428$

+	−9.9431	*	< −0.393− CHG_O_3>	[0.338]
+	7.2334	*	< −0.303− CHG_O_3>	[0.255]
+	0.0233	*	VOLUME	[0.146]
+	5.7143	*	BASICITY	[0.103]
+	−3.3223	*	AMINO_AC	[0.052]
+	−3.5976	*	< −0.395− BASICITY>	[0.046]
+	−1.3567	*	CHG_C_3	[0.028]
+	0.0822	*	<C_AR>	[0.027]

N: 191 LSE: 0.278
LOF: 0.347 r^2: 0.899
r^2_{adj}: 0.895 F: 203.088
SSE: 53.071 SSR: 473.763

FIG. 21. *Model 5 out of 8.*

$\text{LOGP}_{\text{GFA-6}} = 0.843273$

+	−9.964	*	< −0.393− CHG_O_3>	[0.338]
+	7.254	*	< −0.303− CHG_O_3>	[0.256]
+	0.023	*	VOLUME	[0.146]
+	5.715	*	BASICITY	[0.103]
+	−3.322	*	AMINO_AC	[0.052]
+	−3.588	*	< −0.394− BASICITY>	[0.046]
+	−1.356	*	CHG_C_3	[0.028]
+	0.082	*	<C_AR>	[0.027]

N: 191 LSE: 0.278
LOF: 0.347 r^2: 0.899
r^2_{adj}: 0.895 F: 202.944
SSE: 53.105 SSR: 473.730

FIG. 22. *Model 6 out of 8.*

By comparing what is similar and what is different among models in the population, the user can acquire a sense of what kinds of terms are necessary, and which variants are possible.

Model 2 of 8 has a number of differences with the first model. The position of the knots in the CHG_O_3 spline terms are slightly shifted. It contains one linear and one spline use of BASICITY. It uses CHG_C_3 linearly rather than as a spline term. It includes the variable LOG_MW. It uses C_AR as a spline rather than as a linear term. Model 3 of 8 is similar to model 2, but uses two novel terms of the variable CHG_C_AR, one linear and one spline. However, the two terms combined only account for about 5% of the variance of the model, and so the adjustment should be considered minimal.

$\text{LOGP}_{\text{GFA-7}} = -75.679$

+	−181.432	*	BASICITY	[0.3813]
+	−191.275	*	< −0.395− BASICITY>	[0.2883]
+	188.628	*	<BASICITY + 0.393>	[0.2233]
+	−11.548	*	< −0.386− CHG_O_3>	[0.0457]
+	8.099	*	< −0.304− CHG_O_3>	[0.0331]
+	0.025	*	VOLUME	[0.0181]
+	−3.525	*	AMINO_AC	[0.0064]
+	1.472	*	LOG_MW	[0.0035]

N: 191	LSE: 0.285
LOF: 0.347	r^2: 0.897
r^2_{adj}: 0.892	F: 197.352
SSE: 54.454	SSR: 472.380

FIG. 23. *Model 7 out of 8.*

$\text{LOGP}_{\text{GFA-8}} = -5.045$

+	−11.644	*	< −0.386− CHG_O_3>	[0.345]
+	8.685	*	< −0.304− CHG_O_3>	[0.266]
+	0.021	*	VOLUME	[0.115]
+	−9.899	*	< −0.404− BASICITY>	[0.110]
+	6.724	*	<BASICITY + 0.393>	[0.059]
+	−3.523	*	AMINO_AC	[0.048]
+	1.993	*	LOG_MW	[0.035]
+	−0.990	*	CHG_C_3	[0.018]

N: 191	LSE: 0.286
LOF: 0.347	r^2: 0.897
r^2_{adj}: 0.892	F: 196.637
SSE: 54.631	SSR: 473.203

FIG. 24. *Model 8 out of 8.*

Model 4 of 8 is similar to model 2, though it does not use LOG_MW and uses HYDROCAR. CHG_C_3 is used as a spline rather than linearly.

Model 5 of 8 is quite similar to model 2, though it does not use LOG_MW. Model 6 of 8 is the same as model 5, with the one change of a knot position for variable BASICITY.

Models 7 of 8 is quite different. We can notice this by inspecting the coefficients of the BASICITY, which are significantly larger than their values in the other models. This is due to a phenomena called *leverage*; two highly-correlated variables are being used in the model, with large coefficients nearly equal in magnitude but opposite in sign. Usually, such models are discarded, but in this case, the models deserve further inspection. The

$\text{Illumination}_{\text{GFA-1}} = 987$

+	−1693	*	$SrNO_3$	[0.366]
+	−1512	*	$NaNO_3$	[0.327]
+	−12850	*	$< 0.047 - NaNO_3 * SrNO_3 >$	[0.226]
+	3698	*	(Mg * Binder)	[0.078]

N: 15	LSE: 407.9
LOF: 2549	r^2: 0.952
r^2_{adj}: 0.933	F: 49.749
SSE: 6118	SSR: 121754
XV−r^2: 0.90	Full XV−r^2: 0.76

FIG. 25. *Model 1 out of 8.*

$\text{Illumination}_{\text{GFA-2}} = -693$

+	1671	*	Mg	[0.403]
+	−11084	*	$< 0.050 - NaNO_3 * SrNO_3 >$	[0.324]
+	3528	*	Binder	[0.213]
+	410	*	Mg * $NaNO_3$	[0.058]

N: 15	LSE: 413.7
LOF: 2585	r^2: 0.951
r^2_{adj}: 0.932	F: 49.019
SSE: 6205	SSR: 121668

FIG. 26. *Model 2 out of 8.*

spline terms on BASICITY are denoting a subset of the data samples that, by treating as a "special case", can gain a predictive advantage. For model 7, the critical range for BASICITY is $[-0.395, -0.393]$; inspecting the data set, we find 25 compounds, all of which are of the same chemical class: they are all alcohols. The use of "leverage" in model 7 to single out the alcohols and adjust their predictions is unorthodox, but informative. Rejecting or accepting these models is no longer based on the abstract statistical criteria that they contain highly-correlated basis functions, but the domain criteria as to whether alcohols should be treated as a special case in our analysis. If so, this information can be included in the table as an explicit IS_ALCOHOL variable similar to the AMINO_AC variable.

Finally, model 8 of 8 is a curious interpolation between the first 6 models and model 7. The similarity to model 7 is a result of the two spline terms on BASICITY; in this case, however, the range is much larger, covering the region $[-0.404, -0.393]$. Nearly all of the molecules in this region are in one of two classes: alcohols or phenols (aromatic alcohols). The amount of leverage is much smaller, as the more reasonable values of the coefficients testify. The result, however, is the same: the user should

$\text{Illumination}_{\text{GFA-3}} = 924$

+	−1549	*	$SrNO_3$	[0.363]
+	−1368	*	$NaNO_3$	[0.320]
+	−11197	*	$< 0.050 - NaNO_3 * SrNO_3 >$	[0.226]
+	3898	*	(Mg * Binder)	[0.089]

N: 15	LSE: 419.8
LOF: 2624	r^2: 0.951
r^2_{adj}: 0.931	F: 48.261
SSE: 6297	SSR: 121575

FIG. 27. *Model 3 out of 8.*

$\text{Illumination}_{\text{GFA-4}} = -669$

+	1805	*	Mg	[0.412]
+	−12975	*	$< 0.047 - NaNO_3 * SrNO_3 >$	[0.339]
+	3389	*	Binder	[0.193]
+	−396	*	Mg * $SrNO_3$	[0.053]

N: 15	LSE: 428.9
LOF: 2680	r^2: 0.950
r^2_{adj}: 0.930	F: 47.188
SSE: 6433	SSR: 121439

FIG. 28. *Model 4 out of 8.*

recognize this implicit classification of samples, and decide whether to make the suggested category explicit.

By presenting different types of models to the user, the population of models generated by GFA can suggest different possibilities for a a physical interpretation of the data. The exposure of *many* such alternate possibilities, rather than simply being presented with a single so-called "best" model, is of singular advantage to the scientist.

B. The top 8 nonlinear GFA models for Illumination. Details about the top model for Illumination have been discussed elsewhere in the chapter. However, it is worth noting that all of the top 8 models contain a spline term using the product of the concentration of the two salts $NaNO_3$ and $SrNO_3$. Curiously, the spline term is never responsible for most of the variance among the terms of the model; instead, it appears to capture information that allows for increased effectiveness of the linear terms.

Note that there is an implicit constraint on the values of the four concentrations: they must add up to 1.0. That is, (Mg + $NaNO_3$ + $SrNO_3$ + Binder) = 1.0. Some formulations models impose that restriction; GFA requires the user to provide legal samples.

$\text{Illumination}_{\text{GFA-5}} = -594$

+	1671	*	Mg	[0.406]
+	−11306	*	< 0.050− $NaNO_3$ * $SrNO_3$>	[0.333]
+	3349	*	Binder	[0.203]
+	−395	*	Mg * $SrNO_3$	[0.056]

N: 15	LSE: 440.2
LOF: 2751	r^2: 0.948
r^2_{adj}: 0.928	F: 45.907
SSE: 6604	SSR: 121439

FIG. 29. *Model 5 out of 8.*

$\text{Illumination}_{\text{GFA-6}} = -717$

+	1804	*	Mg	[0.435]
+	−12847	*	< 0.047− $NaNO_3$ * $SrNO_3$>	[0.355]
+	3477	*	Binder	[0.209]

N: 15	LSE: 790.8
LOF: 2751	r^2: 0.907
r^2_{adj}: 0.882	F: 35.857
SSE: 11862	SSR: 116010

FIG. 30. *Model 6 out of 8.*

Model 2 is rather difficult to interpret, other than the obvious point that more magnesium is good for brightness.

Model 3 of 8 is identical to model 1 except for the position of the spline knot.

Similarly, model 4 of 8 is closely related to model 2.

Model 5 of 8 is identical to model 4 except for the placement of the spline knot.

Model 6 is interesting, as it postulates linear, positive effects of magnesium and the binder, with a negative effect for the product of the salt concentration. Such "simple" models are often best for scientific interpretation and hypothesis construction with respect to the underlying physical system.

Model 7 of 8 is the same as model 6, with the spline knot shifted.

Finally, model 8 of 8 contains many interaction variables (3 of the 4 terms are interactions). This can make it difficult to interpret, but it could

also be that the system is indeed "interaction driven", and we should hesitate before discarding a model such as this out of hand.

$\text{Illumination}_{\text{GFA-7}} = -642$

+	1671	*	Mg	[0.429]
+	−11197	*	$< 0.050 - NaNO_3 * SrNO_3 >$	[0.349]
+	3437	*	Binder	[0.220]

N: 15	LSE: 800.6
LOF: 2814	r^2: 0.906
r^2_{adj}: 0.880	F: 35.374
SSE: 12009	SSR: 115863

FIG. 31. *Model 7 out of 8.*

$\text{Illumination}_{\text{GFA-8}} =$

+	1574	*	Mg [0.382]	
+	−12783	*	$< 0.047 - NaNO_3 * SrNO_3 >$	[0.356]
+	5650	*	(Mg * Binder)	[0.190]
+	3158	*	($NaNO_3$ * Binder)	[0.071]

N: 15	LSE: 460.7
LOF: 2879	r^2: 0.946
r^2_{adj}: 0.924	F: 43.760
SSE: 6910	SSR: 120962

FIG. 32. *Model 8 out of 8.*

REFERENCES

[1] D. ROGERS AND A.J. HOPFINGER, Application of Genetic Function Approximation (GFA) to Quantitative Structure-Activity Relationships (QSAR) and Quantitative Structure-Property Relationships (QSPR), *Journal of Chemical Information and Computer Science*, **34**, 854–866, 1994.

[2] D. ROGERS, Genetic Function Approximation: A Genetic Approach to Building Quantitative Structure-Activity Models, in *Proceedings of the 10th European Symposium on Quantitative Structure-Activity Relationships: QSAR and Molecular Modeling*, Prous Scientific Publishers, Barcelona, Spain, 1994.

[3] D. ROGERS, Development of the Genetic Function Approximation Algorithm, in *Proceedings of the 6th International Conference on Genetic Algorithms*, San Mateo, CA, Morgan-Kaufmann, 1995.

[4] D. ROGERS, G/SPLINES: A Hybrid of Friedman's Multivariate Adaptive Regression Splines (MARS) Algorithm with Holland's Genetic Algorithm, in *Proceedings of the Fourth International Conference on Genetic Algorithms*, San Diego, Morgan-Kaufmann, San Mateo, July 1991.

[5] D. ROGERS, Data Analysis using G/SPLINES, in *Advances In Neural Processing Systems 4*, Morgan Kaufmann, San Mateo, CA, 1992.

[6] D. FREEDMAN, R. PISANI, R. PURVES, AND ANI ADHIKARI, *Statistics*, W.R. Norton & Co., New York, 2nd Ed., 1991.

[7] S. WOLD, H. WOLD, A. RUHE, W.J. DUNN III, The Colinearity Problem in Linear Regression. The Partial Least Squares (PLS) Approach to Generalized Inverses., *SIAM Journal of Science, Statistics, and Computation*, **5**, 735–743, 1984.

[8] W.G. Glen, W.J. Dunn III, and D.R. Scott, Principal Components Analysis and Partial Least Squares Regression, *Tetrahedron Computer Methodology*, **2**, 279–356, 1989.

[9] D.E. Rumelhart, G.E. Hinton, R.J. Williams, Learning internal representations by error propagation, in *Parallel Distributed Processing: Exploration into the microstructure of cognition*, D.E. Rumelhart, J.L. McClelland, Eds., MIT Press, Cambridge, MA, 1986.

[10] J. Friedman, Multivariate Adaptive Regression Splines, Technical Report No. 102, Laboratory for Computational Statistics, Department of Statistics, Stanford University, November 1988 (revised August 1990).

[11] K.F. Moschner and A. Cece, Development of a General QSAR for Predicting Octanol-Water Partition Coefficients and its Application to Surfactants, in *Environmental Toxicology and Risk Assessment - Third Volume, ASTM STP 1218*, Hughes, J.S., Biddinger, G.R., Mones, E., Eds., American Society for Testing and Materials, Philadelphia, 1995.

[12] D. Rogers, Evolutionary Statistics: Using a Genetic Algorithm and Model Reduction to Isolate Alternate Statistical Hypotheses of Experimental Data, in *Proceedings of the Seventh International Conference on Genetic Algorithms*, Morgan-Kaufmann, San Francisco, 1997.

[13] G. Piepel and J. Cornell, Mixture Experiment Approaches: Examples, Discussion, and Recommendations, *Journal of Quality Technology*, **26**, 3 July 1994.

APPLICATIONS OF DISTRIBUTED COMPUTING TO CONFORMATIONAL SEARCHES

BRIAN T. LUKE*

Abstract. Distributed Computing, as opposed to Parallel Computing, separates the overall goal of the calculation into isolated tasks and performs some or all of the tasks concurrently on different computers. This is very different from the data-parallel computing that is currently performed on shared-memory, or single-image, multiple-processor architectures, and provides an opportunity to try new techniques for problems important to Molecular Modeling and Drug Discovery. In this paper, two applications of distributed computing to conformational searches of molecules are described. The first application finds all low-energy, stable conformations of molecules that show varying degrees of activity as inhibitors of the angiotensin-converting enzyme (ACE). The goal is to find a 3-dimensional arrangement of certain atoms in one or more low-energy conformations of all active inhibitors that are absent from all low-energy conformations of molecules that are inactive. If such an arrangement is found, this putative pharmacophore can be used to test other compounds of unknown activity. The second application of distributed computing is to find the lowest-energy conformation (e.g. the global minimum) for a series of enkephalins; Met-enkephalin, Leu-enkephalin, and (D)Ala(2)-(D)Leu(5)-enkephalin (DADLE). The conformational searches are performed using three different genetic methods; the first is a "standard" Genetic Algorithm (GA) that only marginally qualifies as a distributed program as it is applied here, the second uses Evolutionary Programming (EP) and produces more of a distributed program, and the third uses a Parallel Genetic Algorithm (PGA) which is almost purely a distributed computing procedure.

1. Introduction. In the current Parallel Computing Model, a single task is performed across several processors by distributing the data between the processors, having each processor work on their piece of the data, and then collecting all the results to complete the task. Common implementations of this data-parallel computing model are calculations of the non-bonded energy and derivatives in empirical energy simulations of large biomolecules [1], and the calculations of required integrals in *ab initio* electronic structure calculations [2]. A Distributed Computing Model separates the overall goal of a calculation into independent tasks and performs some or all of these tasks concurrently on different computers. This computing model can also be called task-parallel computing or Network Computing, and the goal is to design an algorithm such that a single computer, or node in the network, performs a large number of calculations compared to the amount of data it has to send to, or receive from, other nodes. In such a case, the program can perform efficiently over a set of nodes connected by a relatively slow medium, such as ethernet using Transmission Communication Protocol/Interrupt Protocol (TCP/IP).

In this report, two different applications of distributed computing are applied to conformational searching problems. The first application [3]

*National Cancer Institute, Frederick Cancer Research and Development Center, P.O. Box B, Frederick, MD 21702-1201.

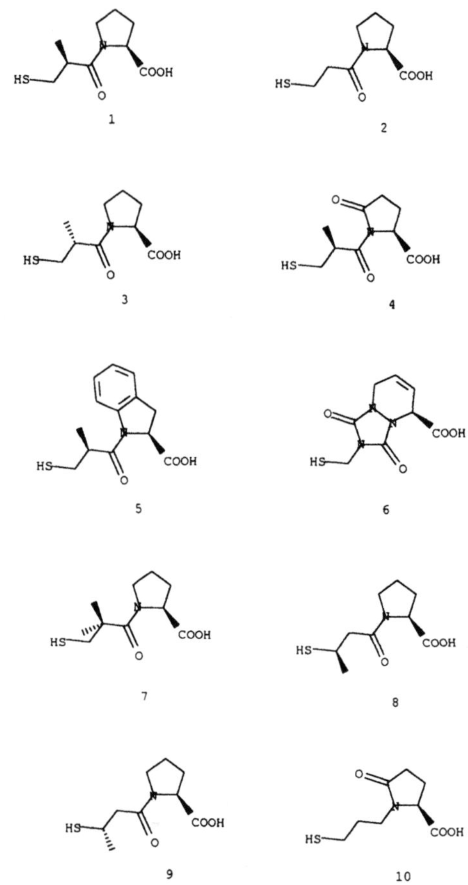

FIG. 1. *The 10 molecules used to find a putative pharmacophore for inhibitors of the angiotensin-converting enzyme (ACE).*

attempts to find a possible pharmacophore for inhibitors of the angiotensin-converting enzyme (ACE). A pharmacophore is defined as the minimum chemical functionality, or 3-dimensional arrangement of specific atoms or groups, a molecule must have in order to exhibit biological activity. This means that different molecules which interact with the same enzymatic receptor site in the same way share a common pharmacophore. If a putative pharmacophore can be determined, it can be used to determine whether untested compounds have a chance of showing biological activity.

The second application [4] uses three different Genetic Methods [5] to search for the lowest energy conformation, e.g. the global minimum, of three different enkephalins; Met-enkephalin, Leu-enkephalin, and (D)Ala(2)-(D)Leu(5)-enkephalin (DADLE). For a molecule with N atoms, the internal, or Potential Energy, is a function of the $3N - 6$ internal degrees of freedom of the molecule. If $1,2$-dichloroethane (Cl-CH_2-CH_2-Cl)

is used as an example, the 3-dimensional conformation of this molecule can be described by 7 bond lengths, 6 bond angles and 5 dihedral angles. The Potential Energy Surface (PES) of this compound represents the internal energy if this molecule for given values of these 18 internal coordinates. Finding the lowest energy point on this PES may appear to be a search in 18-dimensional space, but it actually is only a 1-dimensional problem. Since this molecule only has a single "rotatable" bond, the central C-C bond, only the Cl-C-C-Cl dihedral angle (defined as the angle between the Cl-C-C plane and the C-C-Cl plane, since neither of these bond angles are ever 180°) needs to be scanned. For each value of this dihedral angle, all other internal coordinates can be optimized, producing a 1-dimensional PES.

A similar procedure is used to search for the lowest energy conformation of the three enkephalin analogues. Though finding the lowest energy rigid conformation of flexible polypeptides is not, in itself, crucial to the Drug Discovery process, it can be used for several important purposes. The first is during the development of a method to determine the potential energy for specific conformations of flexible biomolecules. While many development processes attempted to minimize the energy of the experimental conformation, an efficient method of searching conformational space can be used to ensure that the global minimum of the PES is reasonably close to experiment. Another use of the global minimum is in preparing to run Molecular Dynamics or Monte Carlo simulations. For either of these processes, there is always the questions of whether enough simulations have been run, or if they have been run for long enough, to properly sample the PES. If the position of the global minimum on the PES is not known, there is no way to ensure that a sufficient region of conformational space has been sampled. Conversely, if the lowest energy point on the PES is known, it can be used as the starting point from a simulation. This ensures that this energetically favorable region of the PES will be sampled during the simulation(s).

The preceding example also suggests that an efficient search procedure should locate multiple, low-energy conformations of flexible biomolecules, including the global minimum. Each of these conformations can be used as the starting points for subsequent simulations. The genetic methods described below all have the advantage that multiple, low-energy conformations are produced each time the search is run.

The intent of this report is not to simply communicate the results of these studies, but to show how using a distributed computing model can produce new algorithms or new ways of thinking about these problems.

2. Pharmacophore search of ACE inhibitors. Since the structure of ACE is not known, much work has been done to determine stable conformations of known inhibitors, and from them deduce a model for the enzymatic active site [6–9]. The basic hypothesis used in this investigation is that *the conformation of a substrate bound to the active site of an enzyme should be very similar to a low-energy conformation of the free molecule.* Since there will be preferential stabilization of one conformation of a substrate relative to another when it is bound in the active site, there is no way to predict *a priori* which conformation of a particular substrate should be used. Therefore, a collection of conformations should be examined for each possible substrate and the required pharmacophore should be present in at least one low-energy conformation of each active inhibitor and should be missing from all low-energy conformations of inactive compounds.

In this study [3], 10 compounds are examined; these are shown in Figure 1. Compounds **1**–**6** are known to be ACE inhibitors, while Compound **10** is known to be inactive [10]. Compounds **7**–**9** are slight structural modifications of captopril, **1**, and have unknown activities as ACE inhibitors. While previous studies used the semiempirical Austin Model 1 (AM1) Hamiltonian [11] to perform full conformational searches of captopril [12], **1**, and its demethylated analogue [13], **2**, this investigation uses the Parametric Model 3 (PM3) Hamiltonian [14] and a distributed version of Mopac7 [15].

The Mopac7 input file needed to perform a full conformational search of captopril, **1**, is shown in Figure 2. When the distributed version of Mopac7 is run, a *master* process is started and it initiates *slave* processes on N different nodes (though one is usually the same node that is running the master process), where these N nodes are determined by the *hosts* file used when the Parallel Virtual Machine version 3 (PVM3) session is initiated. The master process reads the input file and finds the MULTI keyword on the first line. When the initial geometry is read, six dihedral angles are flagged as "rotatable" bonds by finding a -1 after the value of the dihedral. After the geometry, the master process reads the initial values for each of these rotatable bonds. In this example, the 5-2-1-3 dihedral angle can assume initial values of 0.0 and 180.0°. Similarly, the 13-5-2-1 dihedral angle is able to assume initial values of 60.0, 180.0 and -60.0°. By taking all possible combinations of the initial values for the six rotatable bonds, the master program creates 324 input files. This program then passes the filenames of the first N inputs to the N slave processes, and each slave process optimizes a geometry. When the slave process completes, it notifies the master process and receives the name of a new input file. This procedure continues until all inputs have been processed. By only sending the slave process one input file at a time, a dynamic *load balancing* occurs. This allows the program to run efficiently over nodes with different processor speeds, or over nodes with different loads from other users.

When a geometry optimization completes with the standard version of Mopac7, an input file for the molecular modeling program SYBYL [16] and a Log file are produced along with the normal Archive and Output files. In this distributed version [15], the SYBYL file is not kept unless SYBYL appears on the keyword line, and the Log file is also discarded

```
PM3 MULTI PUSHIT GEO-OK NOLOG NOINPUT MMOK
BUILT FROM capto-i.MOPARC
MULTI OPTIMIZATIONS
N        .00000 0      .00000 0      .00000  0    0   0   0
C       1.41310 1      .00000 0      .00000  0    1   0   0
C       1.48541 1  124.08191 1      .00000  0    1   2   0
C       1.48681 1  123.65839 1  -169.49581  1    1   2   3
C       1.52973 1  117.99829 1   176.51396 -1    2   1   3
O       1.22307 1  117.05503 1   178.67430  1    2   1   5
C       1.53630 1  104.85785 1    13.44606  1    3   1   4
C       1.52635 1  113.77463 1  -120.60197  1    3   1   7
H       1.11964 1  109.55927 1   119.94490  1    3   1   7
C       1.52507 1  106.17526 1    -1.49986  1    4   1   3
H       1.11402 1  108.69965 1   122.46259  1    4   1  10
H       1.11013 1  109.92302 1  -121.77268  1    4   1  10
C       1.52441 1  111.27810 1  -166.18004 -1    5   2   1
C       1.52335 1  109.43123 1  -123.31041  1    5   2  13
H       1.12368 1  107.97697 1   118.17269  1    5   2  13
H       1.10708 1  110.00672 1    99.79498  1    7   3   1
H       1.10500 1  112.33988 1   117.21303  1    7   3  16
O       1.21788 1  126.76771 1  -157.07362 -1    8   3   1
O       1.35178 1  117.81867 1  -178.44551  1    8   3  18
H       1.10512 1  111.32336 1  -132.43056  1   10   4   1
H       1.10603 1  110.79544 1  -117.61309  1   10   4  20
S       1.82946 1  109.02597 1   156.34421 -1   13   5   2
H       1.10549 1  110.55644 1   122.28843  1   13   5  22
H       1.10624 1  110.59596 1  -120.77823  1   13   5  22
H       1.09820 1  110.82325 1   178.17170  1   14   5   2
H       1.10388 1  110.84988 1   119.48995  1   14   5  25
H       1.09769 1  111.93164 1  -120.13390  1   14   5  25
H        .95285 1  109.43390 1  -178.65921 -1   19   8   3
H       1.30769 1   99.09927 1  -178.62341 -1   22  13   5
0 0.0000 0 0.0000 0 0.0000 0 0 0 0
 0.0            180.0
60.0   180.0    -60.0
60.0   180.0    -60.0
60.0   180.0    -60.0
 0.0            180.0
60.0   180.0    -60.0
```

FIG. 2. *Mopac7 MULTI input file to search the conformational space of Captopril (1).*

since the keyword NOLOG is present. To ensure that a local minimum is obtained in the majority of the optimizations, the PUSHIT keyword is also used. This keyword causes the slave process to examine the archive file it has just produced. If the optimization did not converge, the process uses the last geometry to build a new input with the keyword EF (e.g. Eigenvector Following [17]) substituted for PUSHIT, and the optimization is rerun. Finally, to ensure that all of the input files created by the master process are not kept on the user's disk, the NOINPUT keyword is used. This causes the slave process to delete the input file once it has finished with its task.

Since a large number of optimized geometries are obtained for each compound, it is necessary to determine a set of unique, low-energy conformations. This is done by using the program UNIQUE [18], which reads the archive and output files and generates an energy-ordered list of unique conformations. This list of unique conformations for each compound is processed by the program HARVEST [19] to obtain tables of selected internuclear separations, one for each compound. These tables are then used by the program FINDPHARM [20] to search for possible pharmacophores.

In this study, HARVEST determines the internuclear separations between four groups of atoms. Group 1 contains the amide oxygen, and is denoted $C = O$. Group 2 contains the sulfur atom, denoted S, and Group 3 contains the two carboxylic oxygens, denoted [O1,O2]. Group 4 contains the hydrogen that is bound to the sulfur and is denoted $H(S)$. Though many possible pharmacophores can be found for this set of compounds, the results presented here will only describe one analysis by the program FINDPHARM. In this analysis, Compound **6** is used as the "scanning" molecule since it has the smallest number of rotatable bonds and therefore has the fewest number of unique conformations. For each unique conformation of **6** that is within 5.0 kcal/mol of the lowest energy conformation, all possible sets of four internuclear separations are chosen. An error bar of 0.2 Angstroms is added to each separation. This range of four separations must be present in at least one conformation of Compounds **1**–**5** that is within 5.0 kcal/mol of the lowest energy geometry, and absent from all conformations within 5.0 kcal/mol of the lowest geometry in Compound **10**, before it is considered as a possible pharmacophore.

When the results of FINDPHARM are examined, only one set of four distances is found, though it is found multiple times with overlapping ranges. The possible ranges for these distances are

Distance between $C = O$ and $H(S)$ must be between 4.70 and 5.15 Angstroms.

Distance between S and the average coordinate of [O1,O2] must be between 6.96 and 7.46 Angstroms.

Maximum distance between S and [O1,O2] must be between 7.72 and 8.28 Angstroms.

Minimum distance between S and [O1,O2] must be between 6.26 and 6.74 Angstroms.

Conformations satisfying these conditions are found for one conformation of **1**, three conformations of **2**, five conformations of **3**, three conformations of **4**, four conformations of **5**, five conformations of **6**, one conformation of **7**, and no low-energy conformations of **8–10**. If these ranges of internuclear separations represent the required pharmacophore for ACE inhibitors, these results suggest that Compound **7** may show some activity, while Compounds **8** and **9** should show no activity as ACE inhibitors. If these predictions are not correct, some other combination of internuclear separations might be important but was not examined here, or it may be that only a set of three internuclear separations is necessary to describe the pharmacophore. The latter possibility would be unfortunate since an analysis using only three sets of internuclear separations produces a large number of possible pharmacophores.

3. Conformational searches of flexible polypeptides using genetic methods. This study uses a Genetic Algorithm, Evolutionary Programming, and a Parallel Genetic Algorithm to search for the global minimum of the potential energy surface for Met-enkephalin, Leu-enkephalin, and DADLE using the Empirical Conformational Energy Program for Peptides, version 2 (ECEPP/2) [21]. The ECEPP/2 global minimum of Met-enkephalin is a good test since this structure has been previously found using three different search techniques [22–24].

Each of these genetic methods are "guided stochastic" search procedures, though differ from other strategies (such as Simulated Annealing) in that a relatively large number of conformations are stored by the program, and can be thought of as representing "animals" in a population. These conformations will be used to create new conformations, or "offspring", and a "survival of the fittest" strategy will be used to determine which conformations remain in the population and which are discarded.

The first step is to determine how a conformation will be represented in the program. Met-enkephalin, for example, has 24 "rotatable" bonds. By setting these dihedral angles to specific values, the 3-dimensional structure of this penta-peptide is completely determined. Therefore, a particular conformation in a group of NPOP conformation is represented by a Genetic Vector [4] that contains 24 real numbers between 0.0 and 360.0° (giving the values of these 24 dihedral angles).

Instead of attempting to maximize the fitness of a particular animal, these procedures will try to minimize the cost of a conformation. In this study, the cost is simply the energy of that conformation as determined by the ECEPP/2 empirical energy potential. Before the results of the searches are presented, a brief overview of how Genetic Algorithms, Evolutionary Programming, and a Parallel Genetic Algorithm can be applied to this problem will be given, with a special emphasis on how they can be used in a Distributed Computing environment.

Genetic Algorithm

In a Genetic Algorithm [25], new conformations of the penta-peptides (called *offspring*) are created by taking pieces of the Genetic Vector from two conformations (called *parents*) in the current population, and is denoted a *mating operation.* The general flow of the genetic algorithm [26] used in this study is as follows.

1. Generate an initial population of *NPOP* conformations. In this study, two different techniques are used. The first is to use a random number generator to determine initial dihedral angles for each of the rotatable bonds, except for the omega-angles which are initially fixed at 180°. Each structure is then optimized. This technique is denoted AUTO. The second technique uses conformations that are created by the program PEPTOR [28]. PEPTOR finds low-energy conformations of polpeptides by performing full scans of torsional space for each rotatable bond, selected in different orders. This method of generating the initial population will be denoted PEPTOR.

2. Select two *parents* from the current population for mating. In this implementation [26], one of the parents is chosen randomly and the other is chosen based upon its fitness. This differs from other implementations that use a *mating pool* [4], which causes both parents to be chosen based upon their fitness, or algorithms that promote *niching* by selecting the second parent based upon its similarity to the first. Two different techniques are used to perform the fitness-based selection of the second parent. The first orders the solutions in the current population from best to worst (lowest to highest energy) and selects the number of the parent, I, from the equation

$$I = NPOP^*\{A - SQRT[A^2 - 4.0^*(A - 1.0)^*RAN]\}/[2.0^*(A - 1.0)]$$

where RAN is a random number between 0.0 and 1.0 [27]. A is a user-defined parameter that must be greater than 1.0. As the value of A increases, so does the probability that the number of the parent will be closer to 1, meaning that a lower-energy conformation in the current population will be chosen as a parent. The denotation for this selection process is to list the value for A, and in this example, values of 2.0 and 2.5 are used. The second technique takes this selection to the obvious extreme; the lowest-energy (dominant) conformation in the current population is always used as the second parent. This technique is denoted *Dom.*

3. Use a mating operator to initially generate one or more offspring. This operator combines the genetic vectors of the two parents to create a genetic vector for an offspring. The standard procedure is to choose a place along the genetic vector and cut the genetic vectors of each parent at this point. The offspring is created by using the first sub-vector from one parent and the second sub-vector from the other. Such a mating operator is called a *single-point crossover*. In this study, an *unbiased uniform crossover* [4] is used. This means that each torsion angle (gene) is randomly selected from one or the other parent.

4. Use a mutation operator to slightly change some of the dihedral angles in the genetic vector. As with most applications of genetic algorithms [4,25], the mutation operator plays a very minor role. In this implementation, a small, random amount is added to, or subtracted from, the torsion angle for a few randomly chosen genes in the genetic vector of an offspring.

5. Optimize the conformation of each offspring. This *maturation operator* is found to greatly increase the convergence of the algorithm to good solutions, and is particularly necessary since each gene in the genetic vector can assume an infinite number of values (all real numbers between 0.0 and 360.0). If the dihedral angles were forced to assume only integer values, the parameter space would become finite and maturation may not be as necessary, though it still would speed up the convergence rate. The cost of each offspring is equal to the energy at this minimum.

6. Update the population. In this application, several offspring are created from each pair of parents and optimized. The lowest energy offspring replaces the higher-energy parent in the population. This is different than the standard implementation of a genetic algorithm, where the offspring replaces the weakest member in the entire population. Tests suggest that this latter replacement procedure accelerates the convergence of genetic algorithms by increasing the rate of forming *schema* [4], which means that all solutions in the current population contain the same value for a particular element in the genetic vector, but also increases the chance of converging to a sub-optimal conformation. One possible reason for this is that all genetic information (dihedral angles) contained in the genetic vector of the least fit solution in the population is lost after each mating and is replaced by a solution that should have some similarity to its parents. In the procedure used here, each conformation in the population has the opportunity to pass potentially good genes to an offspring before it is removed from the population.

In this implementation, the program is not well designed for a network computing environment. The main reason is that the best offspring replaces a member of the current population, which means that this offspring can be one of the parents in the very next mating. Such an algorithm is denoted *nongenerational* [4]. If the offspring were placed into a new population, this would become a *generational* algorithm that would run efficiently on a network of compute nodes. Each node would be given a parent pair and they would use mating and mutation operators to generate multiple offspring. Each offspring would be allowed to maturate, and the lowest-energy offspring would be placed into the new population. When NPOP offspring are present in this new population, the next generation's parent population can be constructed by either using the new population or choosing NPOP solutions from the old and new populations using either a *deterministic* or *probabilistic* procedure, with or without evoking an *elitist strategy* [4].

When the results of a genetic algorithm search are compared to those generated by the other methods, a particular run will be denoted *GA/Sel*

(Noff) where *Sel* denotes the procedure used to select the second parent (and would be either 2.0, 2.5 or *Dom*) and *Noff* is the number of offspring examined for each mating pair. Therefore, *GA/Dom(10)* means that the Genetic Algorithm always uses the dominant conformation as one of the parents and 10 offspring are created and minimized, with the lowest-energy conformation replacing the weaker parent.

Evolutionary Programming

In this chapter, the term "evolutionary methods" is used to denote methods that differ from Genetic methods in that the offspring are generated by *asexual reproduction*. In other words, only a single parent is used to generate an offspring with the aid of a mutation operator. This class of methods includes Evolutionary Programming [29], Evolutionary Strategies [30], and their variants [4]. The general flow of the evolutionary method used in this study is as follows.

1. Generate an initial population of *NPOP* conformations. As with the genetic algorithm, this study uses two different techniques. *AUTO* uses a random number generator to determine initial dihedral angles for each of the rotatable bonds, except for the omega-angles which are initially fixed at 180°. Each structure is then optimized. The second technique, *PEPTOR*, uses conformations that are created by the program *PEPTOR* [28].

2. Each conformation in the current population is used to generate a single offspring. All values of the dihedral angles are initially copied from the parent to this offspring. Three dihedral angles (not necessarily different) are then chosen at random. If the selected angle is not an omega-angle, it is set to a random value between 0.0 and 360.0°. Omega-angles are set to a random value between 150.0 and 210.0°. This structure is minimized and placed into a new population, meaning that a *generational* algorithm is used.

3. A *deterministic* updating procedure [4] is used to determine the parent population for the next generation. This means that the best *NPOP* conformations are chosen from the parent and offspring populations.

Since a generational algorithm is used, this procedure can be effectively run on a network of CPUs. A master process sequentially passes the genetic vector of each parent to slave processes running on different nodes. Each slave process generates an offspring through mutation, optimizes its geometry, and passes the final genetic vector and cost (minimized energy) back to the master process. When all parents have generated an offspring, the master process selects the best *NPOP* conformations and a generation is complete. Since each slave process only receives one parent at a time, a dynamic load balancing is achieved.

Since no selection procedure is used (all parents are used each generation) and only a single offspring is generated, the results of an Evolutionary Programming run will simply be denoted *EP* in the tables of results. Different *EP* runs on the same polypeptide will only differ from each other by the way the initial population is generated (*AUTO* versus *PEPTOR*) and the seed to the random number generator.

Parallel Genetic Algorithm

The Parallel Genetic Algorithm [4,31], PGA, used here should actually be called a Distributed Genetic Algorithm since a separate population of *NPOP* solutions is processed on different nodes of a workstation cluster. The general flow of the PGA used in this study is as follows.

1. *NPOP* conformations are automatically created (randomly assigned initial values and optimized) on each of *NODES* nodes of the cluster.
2. Multiple offspring are created from each parent pair using the same selection, mating and mutation operators that are used for the standard GA described above. After optimization, the lowest-energy offspring replaces the higher-energy parent in the population. A "generation" is complete when *NPOP* offspring have been placed in the population.
3. After *NGEN* generations, the best conformation from each population is copied to an adjacent node in a ring orientation, where it replaces the weakest member of the population.
4. This process is then repeated *NTOT* times.

A PGA uses the strength of a standard genetic algorithm (the formation of schema to reduce the dimensionality of the search space) and allows each population to independently converge on various regions of conformational space. By seeding each population with a good solution from another, the hope is to occasionally shock a population with new genes so that it does not converge on a sub-optimal solution.

Though this algorithm is distributed by design, it can suffer from load balancing problems since every *NGEN* generations the process must stop and wait until all nodes are ready to pass a conformation to one node and receive a conformation from another. This means that each "cycle" in this process can only proceed at the rate of the slowest node in the network.

When PGA results are compared to those obtained by the other methods, the following notation will be used; *PGA/Sel-NODES-NPOP-NTOT-NGEN(Noff)*, where *Sel* denotes the procedure used to select the second parent (and would be either 2.0, 2.5 or *Dom*), *NODES* is the number of nodes (populations) used, *NPOP* is the population size on each node, *NGEN* is the number of generations each node goes through before a conformation is passed to, and received from, another population, *NTOT* is the number of times this process is repeated, and *Noff* is the number of offspring examined for each mating pair. Therefore, *PGA/2.0-8-20-16-5(3)* means that 8 nodes are used with a population of 20 conformations on each node. The parent selection procedure uses a biasing value of 2.0 to select one parent (the other is randomly chosen) and 3 offspring are created and optimized for each parent pair (the weaker parent is replaced by the most-fit offspring). This procedure is run for 5 "generations" and the lowest

TABLE 1

Energies (kcal/mol) for the lowest-energy conformation of Met-enkephalin using three runs (R-1 through R-3) of a Genetic Algorithm and Evolutionary Programming.[a]

Method	Source[b]	R-1	R-2	R-3
GA/Dom(10)	PEPTOR	-16.1	-16.1	-16.1
GA/2.5(10)	PEPTOR	-16.1	-16.1	-16.1
GA/2.0(10)	PEPTOR	-16.1	-16.1	-16.1
GA/Dom(10)	AUTO	-16.1	-14.4	-16.1
GA/2.5(10)	AUTO	-16.0	-14.3	-16.1
GA/2.0(10)	AUTO	-14.0	-12.7	-16.0
EP	PEPTOR	-16.1	-16.1	-16.1
EP	AUTO	-16.1	-16.1	-12.2

[a]The three runs differ only in the seed for the random number generator. For R-1 through R-3, they are 837457, 3837457, and 7837457, respectively.
[b]This column gives the source of the initial conformations.

energy conformation is passed to the next node in a ring orientation. This process is repeated 16 times.

The results for conformational searches of Met-enkephalin are shown in Table 1 using GA and EP methods. These results show that the global minimum (with an energy of approximately -16.1 kcal/mol [24]) is found the majority of the time. The GA finds this structure all 9 times when the initial population is obtained from the program PEPTOR, and 5 of the 9 times when the initial population is randomly generated. The EP search finds the global minimum all 3 times when the initial population is determined by PEPTOR, and 2 out of 3 times when the initial population is randomly generated. Since these methods consistently find the global minimum, a PGA search has not been attempted.

The results for conformational searches of Leu-enkephalin are shown in Table 2 for all three search methods. A final conformation with an energy of -14.2 kcal/mol or less is found 8 times. The GA did not find a conformation at or below this energy in any of the 30 runs. EP found conformations at or below this energy in 2 of the 10 runs, and the PGA found conformations in 6 of the 15 runs. These 8 structures yield 2 unique conformations. Conformation-1 contains the 2 EP results and the 3 PGA conformations with an energy of -14.4 kcal/mol. Conformation-2 contains the PGA structures with energies of -14.2 and -14.3 kcal/mol. There is approximately a 70% similarity [32] between these conformations. Since these searches produce one or more final populations of results, it is possible that Conformation-2 is also found in the runs that find Conformation-1.

The conformational search results for (D)Ala(2)-(D)Leu(5)-enkephalin show that a final conformation of -12.0 kcal/mol or less is found 8 times. The GA did not find any in the 18 runs, EP finds 3 conformations in 6 runs,

TABLE 2

Energies (kcal/mol) for the lowest-energy conformation of Leu-enkephalin using five runs (R-1 through R-5) of a Genetic Algorithm, Evolutionary Programming, and a Parallel Genetic Algorithm.[a]

Method	**Source**[b]	**R-1**	**R-2**	**R-3**	**R-4**	**R-5**
GA/Dom(10)	PEPTOR	-10.7	-12.7	-12.9	-11.4	-12.9
GA/2.5(10)	PEPTOR	-13.0	-13.0	-13.1	-12.7	-12.9
GA/2.0(10)	PEPTOR	-12.8	-12.9	-12.9	-12.9	-10.6
GA/Dom(10)	AUTO	-13.4	-13.0	-12.9	-13.0	-11.1
GA/2.5(10)	AUTO	-13.0	-13.1	-13.1	-12.9	-13.6
GA/2.0(10)	AUTO	-13.0	-13.1	-13.0	-13.0	-12.9
EP	PEPTOR	-12.8	-14.3	-13.3	-13.1	-14.4
EP	AUTO	-13.1	-13.1	-13.1	-13.1	-13.1
PGA/Dom-8-20-16-5(3)	AUTO	-13.5	-13.0	-14.4	-12.9	-14.3
PGA/2.5-8-20-16-5(3)	AUTO	-13.2	-14.2	-14.4	-13.1	-14.4
PGA/2.0-8-20-16-5(3)	AUTO	-13.1	-13.1	-13.1	-14.2	-13.4

[a] The five runs differ only in the seed for the random number generator. For R-1 through R-5, they are 837457, 3837457, 7837457, 17837457, and 27837457, respectively.

[b] This column gives the source of the initial conformations.

and the PGA finds a conformation in 7 of 9 runs. These 10 structures yield 3 unique conformations. Conformation-1 contains the 2 PGA structures with energies of -12.3 and -12.4 kcal/mol. Conformation-2 contains all 7 structures with an energy of -12.1 kcal/mol (3 EP and 4 PGA), and it has a 33% similarity to Conformation-1. Conformation-3 is the PGA structure with an energy of -12.0 kcal/mol. This conformation has a 67% similarity with Conformation-1 and a 37% similarity with Conformation-2. Again, since multiple conformations are produced in each run, Conformation-2 may also be present in the runs that find Conformation-1, and Conformation-3 may be present in the final population(s) that find either Conformation-1 or Conformation-2.

4. Conclusions. Both of the studies outlined above strongly suggest that a conformational search algorithm should be torsion-angle driven. The procedures described above have been used with the semiempirical PM3 Hamiltonian and the ECEPP/2 empirical energy potential, but can be used with any force field or level of theory. In searches for the global minimum of three different enkephalins, the results presented above suggest that, *as used here*, the Parallel Genetic Algorithm performs the best, followed by Evolutionary Programming and a standard Genetic Algorithm. Different choices of the population size, number of generations, mating/mutation operators, or the form of the genetic vector can affect the final results obtained by these methods.

TABLE 3

Energies (kcal/mol) for the lowest-energy conformation of (D)Ala(2)-(D)Leu(5)-enkephalin using three runs (R-1 through R-3) of a Genetic Algorithm, Evolutionary Programming, and a Parallel Genetic Algorithm.[a]

Method	Source[b]	R-1	R-2	R-3
GA/Dom(10)	PEPTOR	-7.9	-7.9	-7.9
GA/2.5(10)	PEPTOR	-8.7	-7.9	-7.9
GA/2.0(10)	PEPTOR	-7.9	-7.9	-7.9
GA/Dom(10)	AUTO	-9.0	-11.0	-8.8
GA/2.5(10)	AUTO	-9.1	-10.0	-11.4
GA/2.0(10)	AUTO	-11.8	-11.0	-11.1
EP	PEPTOR	-12.1	-12.1	-9.1
EP	AUTO	-11.1	-12.1	-11.1
PGA/Dom-8-20-16-5(3)	AUTO	-11.8	-12.4	-12.1
PGA/2.5-8-20-16-5(3)	AUTO	-11.6	-12.1	-12.0
PGA/2.0-8-20-16-5(3)	AUTO	-12.1	-12.3	-12.1

[a] The three runs differ only in the seed for the random number generator. For R-1 through R-3, they are 837457, 3837457, and 7837457, respectively.
[b] This column gives the source of the initial conformations.

By adopting a distributed computing model, several procedures have been presented that can aid in the search for pharmacophores or search for the lowest-energy conformation of flexible molecules. It should be stressed that these are simply new ways to examine existing problems, and should be taken as new tools in the toolbox of methods available to computational chemists. No single method should be adopted as *the* way to search the conformational space of a molecule or else researchers may be forced to adopt the "Hammer Principle". This principle simply states that if a hammer is the only tool available in a toolbox, everything begins to look like a nail. A more mathematical treatment of this principle can be found in the "No Free Lunch Theorems for Search" [33]. Here, the authors demonstrate that in the uncountably-infinite number of optimization problems available, a single method is only able to solve a finite, or countably-infinite, number of them. This means that any single search method solves 0% of the total number, and if a researcher uses only one method for all problems, it might as well be a "random guess," since this method is very fast and has the same probability of finding all solutions as any other method. A final way to state this is simply that the problem should dictate which search procedures to use, not the other way around.

REFERENCES

[1] J.F. JANIK AND P.C. PATTNAIK, J. Comput. Chem. 13 (1992) 533;
S.L. LIN, J. MELLOR-CRUMMEY, B.M. PETTITT AND G.N. PHILLIPS, JR., J. Comput. Chem. 13 (1992) 1022;
S.E. DEBOLT AND P.A. KOLLMAN, J. Comput. Chem. 14 (1993) 312.

[2] H.P. LUTHI, J.E. MERTS, M.W. FEYEREISEN AND J.E. ALMLOF, J. Comput. Chem. 13 (1992) 160;
S. KINDERMANN, E. MICHEL AND P. OTTO, J. Comput. Chem. 13 (1992) 414;
M.F. GUEST, P. SHERWOOD AND J.H. VAN LENTHE, Theor. Chim. Acta 84 (1993) 423.

[3] B.T. LUKE, http://members.aol.com/btluke/acepapl.htm.

[4] B.T. LUKE, in *PRINCIPLES IN QSAR AND DRUG DESIGN, VOLUME 1: Genetic Algorithms in Molecular Modeling*, J. Devillers (ed), Academic Press Ltd., London (1996), Ch. 2;
B.T. LUKE, http://members.aol.com/btluke/gmovrl.htm.

[5] B.T. LUKE, http://members.aol.com/btluke/enkephl.htm.

[6] P.R. ANDREWS, J.M. CARSON, A. CASSELI, M.J. SPARK AND R. WOODS, J. Med. Chem., 28 (1985) 393.

[7] R.E. GALARDY AND D. GROBELNY, J. Med. Chem. 28 (1985) 1422.

[8] E.D. THORSETT, E.E. HARRIS, S. ASTER, E.R. PETERSON, J.P. SNYDER, J. HIRSHFIELD, E.W. TRISTRAM, A.A. PATCHETT, E.H. ULM AND T.C. VASSIL, J. Med. Chem. 29 (1986) 251.

[9] D. MEYER, C.B. NAYLOR, I. MOTOC AND G.R. MARSHALL, J. Comput. Aid. Mol. Des. 1 (1987) 3.

[10] E.D. THORSETT, E.E. HARRIS, S.D. ASTER, E.R. PETERSON, J.P. SNYDER, J.P. SPRINGER, J. HIRSCHFIELD, E.W. TRISTRAM, A.A. PATCHETT, E.H. ULM AND T.C. VASSIL, J. Med. Chem. 29 (1986) 251.

[11] M.J.S. DEWAR, E.G. ZOEBISCH, E.F. HEALY AND J.J.P. STEWART, J. Am. Chem. Soc., 107 (1985) 3902;
The sulfur parameters are taken from AMPAC, Version 2.1, M.J.S. Dewar, E.F. HEALY, D.A. LIOTARD AND J.M. RUIS, Quantum Chemistry Program Exchange, Indiana University, Bloomington, IN, Program Number 506.

[12] B.T. LUKE, J. Mol. Struct. (Theochem) 309 (1995) 1.

[13] B.T. LUKE, J. Mol. Struct. (Theochem) 332 (1995) 25.

[14] J.J.P. STEWART, J. Comp. Chem. 10 (1989) 221.

[15] B.T. LUKE, Modified Mopac7 (IBMWS/PVM3) by J.J.P. Stewart et. al, Quantum Chemistry Program Exchange, Indiana University, Bloomington, IN, 1994;
B.T. LUKE, http://members.aol.com/btluke/mopac7.htm.

[16] SYBYL is a registered trademark of Tripos, Inc., 1699 S. Hanley Road, St. Louis, MO 63144-2913.

[17] J. BAKER, J. Comput. Chem. 7 (1986) 385.

[18] B.T. LUKE, http://members.aol.com/btluke/uniquel.htm.

[19] B.T. LUKE, http://members.aol.com/btluke/harvest.htm.

[20] B.T. LUKE, http://members.aol.com/btluke/findph.htm.

[21] F.A. MOMANY, R.F. MCGUIRE, A.W. BURGESS AND H.A. SCHERAGA, J. Phys. Chem. 79 (1975) 2361;
G. NEMETHY, M.S. POTTLE AND H.A. SCHERAGA, J. Phys. Chem. 87 (1983) 1883;
H.A. SCHERAGA et. al, Quantum Chemistry Program Exchange, Indiana University, Bloomington, IN, Program Number 558.

[22] Z. LI AND H.A. SCHERAGA, J. Mol. Struct. (Theochem) 179 (1988) 333; Proc. Natl. Acad. Sci. (U.S.A.) 84 (1987) 6611.

[23] E.O. PURISIMA AND H.A. SCHERAGA, J. Mol. Biol. 196 (1987) 697.

[24] B.T. LUKE, http://members.aol.com/btluke/fold01.htm.

[25] H.J. BREMREMANN, "Numerical Optimization Procedures Derived from Biological Evolution Processes" in Cybernetic Problems in Bionics, H.L. OESTREICHER

AND D.R. MOORE (eds), Gordon and Breach, New York (1968);
J.H. HOLLAND, Adaptation in Natural and Artificial Systems, University of Michigan Press, Ann Arbor (1975);
D.E. GOLDBERG, Genetic Algorithms in Search, Optimization and Machine Learning, Addison-Wesley, Reading, MA (1989);
W. LINERT, P. MARGL AND E. NUSTERER, Computers Chem. 15 (1991) 1.

[26] B.T. LUKE, http://members.aol.com/btluke/genopt1.htm.

[27] D. WHITLEY, Proc. Third Internat. Conf. on Genetic Algorithms, J.D. SCHAFFER (ed), (Morgan Kaufmann, Los Altos, CA, 1989) 166.

[28] B.T. LUKE, http://members.aol.com/btluke/peptor1.htm.

[29] L.J. FOGEL, A/J. OWENS AND M.J. WALSH, Artificial Intelligence through Simulated Evolution, John Wiley, New York (1966);
D.B. FOGEL, Cybern. Syst. 24 (1993) 27.

[30] I. RECHENBERG, Evolutionsstrategie: Optimierung technischer Systeme nach Prinsipien der Biologischen Evolution, Frommann-Holzboog Verlag, Stuttgart (1973);
H.-P. SCHWEFEL, Interdisciplinary Systems Research, Volume 26, Birkhauser, Basel (1977).

[31] H. MUHLENBEIN, M. SCHOMISCH AND J. BORN, Parallel Computing 17 (1991) 619.

[32] B.T. LUKE, SIMBIG (IBMWS/PVM3), Quantum Chemistry Program Exchange, Indiana University, Bloomington, IN, 1994;
B.T. LUKE, http://members.aol.com/btluke/simbig1.htm.

[33] D.H. WOLPERT AND W.G. MACREADY, ftp://ftp.santafe.edu/pub/wgm/nfl.ps.

IMA SUMMER PROGRAMS

1987 Robotics
1988 Signal Processing
1989 Robust Statistics and Diagnostics
1990 Radar and Sonar (June 18 - June 29)
New Directions in Time Series Analysis (July 2 - July 27)
1991 Semiconductors
1992 Environmental Studies: Mathematical, Computational, and Statistical Analysis
1993 Modeling, Mesh Generation, and Adaptive Numerical Methods for Partial Differential Equations
1994 Molecular Biology
1995 Large Scale Optimizations with Applications to Inverse Problems, Optimal Control and Design, and Molecular and Structural Optimization
1996 Emerging Applications of Number Theory (July 15 – July 26)
Theory of Random Sets (August 22 – August 24)
1997 Statistics in the Health Sciences
1998 Coding and Cryptography (July 6 – July 18)
Mathematical Modeling in Industry (July 22 – July 31)

SPRINGER LECTURE NOTES FROM THE IMA:

The Mathematics and Physics of Disordered Media
Editors: Barry Hughes and Barry Ninham
(Lecture Notes in Math., Volume 1035, 1983)

Orienting Polymers
Editor: J.L. Ericksen
(Lecture Notes in Math., Volume 1063, 1984)

New Perspectives in Thermodynamics
Editor: James Serrin
(Springer-Verlag, 1986)

Models of Economic Dynamics
Editor: Hugo Sonnenschein
(Lecture Notes in Econ., Volume 264, 1986)

The IMA Volumes in Mathematics and its Applications

Current Volumes:

1 **Homogenization and Effective Moduli of Materials and Media** J. Ericksen, D. Kinderlehrer, R. Kohn, and J.-L. Lions (eds.)
2 **Oscillation Theory, Computation, and Methods of Compensated Compactness** C. Dafermos, J. Ericksen, D. Kinderlehrer, and M. Slemrod (eds.)
3 **Metastability and Incompletely Posed Problems** S. Antman, J. Ericksen, D. Kinderlehrer, and I. Muller (eds.)
4 **Dynamical Problems in Continuum Physics** J. Bona, C. Dafermos, J. Ericksen, and D. Kinderlehrer (eds.)
5 **Theory and Applications of Liquid Crystals** J. Ericksen and D. Kinderlehrer (eds.)
6 **Amorphous Polymers and Non-Newtonian Fluids** C. Dafermos, J. Ericksen, and D. Kinderlehrer (eds.)
7 **Random Media** G. Papanicolaou (ed.)
8 **Percolation Theory and Ergodic Theory of Infinite Particle Systems** H. Kesten (ed.)
9 **Hydrodynamic Behavior and Interacting Particle Systems** G. Papanicolaou (ed.)
10 **Stochastic Differential Systems, Stochastic Control Theory, and Applications** W. Fleming and P.-L. Lions (eds.)
11 **Numerical Simulation in Oil Recovery** M.F. Wheeler (ed.)
12 **Computational Fluid Dynamics and Reacting Gas Flows** B. Engquist, M. Luskin, and A. Majda (eds.)
13 **Numerical Algorithms for Parallel Computer Architectures** M.H. Schultz (ed.)
14 **Mathematical Aspects of Scientific Software** J.R. Rice (ed.)
15 **Mathematical Frontiers in Computational Chemical Physics** D. Truhlar (ed.)
16 **Mathematics in Industrial Problems** A. Friedman
17 **Applications of Combinatorics and Graph Theory to the Biological and Social Sciences** F. Roberts (ed.)
18 ***q*-Series and Partitions** D. Stanton (ed.)
19 **Invariant Theory and Tableaux** D. Stanton (ed.)
20 **Coding Theory and Design Theory Part I: Coding Theory** D. Ray-Chaudhuri (ed.)
21 **Coding Theory and Design Theory Part II: Design Theory** D. Ray-Chaudhuri (ed.)
22 **Signal Processing Part I: Signal Processing Theory** L. Auslander, F.A. Grünbaum, J.W. Helton, T. Kailath, P. Khargonekar, and S. Mitter (eds.)

23 **Signal Processing Part II: Control Theory and Applications of Signal Processing** L. Auslander, F.A. Grünbaum, J.W. Helton, T. Kailath, P. Khargonekar, and S. Mitter (eds.)

24 **Mathematics in Industrial Problems, Part 2** A. Friedman

25 **Solitons in Physics, Mathematics, and Nonlinear Optics** P.J. Olver and D.H. Sattinger (eds.)

26 **Two Phase Flows and Waves** D.D. Joseph and D.G. Schaeffer (eds.)

27 **Nonlinear Evolution Equations that Change Type** B.L. Keyfitz and M. Shearer (eds.)

28 **Computer Aided Proofs in Analysis** K. Meyer and D. Schmidt (eds.)

29 **Multidimensional Hyperbolic Problems and Computations** A. Majda and J. Glimm (eds.)

30 **Microlocal Analysis and Nonlinear Waves** M. Beals, R. Melrose, and J. Rauch (eds.)

31 **Mathematics in Industrial Problems, Part 3** A. Friedman

32 **Radar and Sonar, Part I** R. Blahut, W. Miller, Jr., and C. Wilcox

33 **Directions in Robust Statistics and Diagnostics: Part I** W.A. Stahel and S. Weisberg (eds.)

34 **Directions in Robust Statistics and Diagnostics: Part II** W.A. Stahel and S. Weisberg (eds.)

35 **Dynamical Issues in Combustion Theory** P. Fife, A. Liñán, and F.A. Williams (eds.)

36 **Computing and Graphics in Statistics** A. Buja and P. Tukey (eds.)

37 **Patterns and Dynamics in Reactive Media** H. Swinney, G. Aris, and D. Aronson (eds.)

38 **Mathematics in Industrial Problems, Part 4** A. Friedman

39 **Radar and Sonar, Part II** F.A. Grünbaum, M. Bernfeld, and R.E. Blahut (eds.)

40 **Nonlinear Phenomena in Atmospheric and Oceanic Sciences** G.F. Carnevale and R.T. Pierrehumbert (eds.)

41 **Chaotic Processes in the Geological Sciences** D.A. Yuen (ed.)

42 **Partial Differential Equations with Minimal Smoothness and Applications** B. Dahlberg, E. Fabes, R. Fefferman, D. Jerison, C. Kenig, and J. Pipher (eds.)

43 **On the Evolution of Phase Boundaries** M.E. Gurtin and G.B. McFadden

44 **Twist Mappings and Their Applications** R. McGehee and K.R. Meyer (eds.)

45 **New Directions in Time Series Analysis, Part I** D. Brillinger, P. Caines, J. Geweke, E. Parzen, M. Rosenblatt, and M.S. Taqqu (eds.)

46 **New Directions in Time Series Analysis, Part II**
D. Brillinger, P. Caines, J. Geweke, E. Parzen, M. Rosenblatt, and M.S. Taqqu (eds.)

47 **Degenerate Diffusions**
W.-M. Ni, L.A. Peletier, and J.-L. Vazquez (eds.)

48 **Linear Algebra, Markov Chains, and Queueing Models**
C.D. Meyer and R.J. Plemmons (eds.)

49 **Mathematics in Industrial Problems, Part 5** A. Friedman

50 **Combinatorial and Graph-Theoretic Problems in Linear Algebra**
R.A. Brualdi, S. Friedland, and V. Klee (eds.)

51 **Statistical Thermodynamics and Differential Geometry of Microstructured Materials**
H.T. Davis and J.C.C. Nitsche (eds.)

52 **Shock Induced Transitions and Phase Structures in General Media** J.E. Dunn, R. Fosdick, and M. Slemrod (eds.)

53 **Variational and Free Boundary Problems**
A. Friedman and J. Spruck (eds.)

54 **Microstructure and Phase Transitions**
D. Kinderlehrer, R. James, M. Luskin, and J.L. Ericksen (eds.)

55 **Turbulence in Fluid Flows: A Dynamical Systems Approach**
G.R. Sell, C. Foias, and R. Temam (eds.)

56 **Graph Theory and Sparse Matrix Computation**
A. George, J.R. Gilbert, and J.W.H. Liu (eds.)

57 **Mathematics in Industrial Problems, Part 6** A. Friedman

58 **Semiconductors, Part I**
W.M. Coughran, Jr., J. Cole, P. Lloyd, and J. White (eds.)

59 **Semiconductors, Part II**
W.M. Coughran, Jr., J. Cole, P. Lloyd, and J. White (eds.)

60 **Recent Advances in Iterative Methods**
G. Golub, A. Greenbaum, and M. Luskin (eds.)

61 **Free Boundaries in Viscous Flows**
R.A. Brown and S.H. Davis (eds.)

62 **Linear Algebra for Control Theory**
P. Van Dooren and B. Wyman (eds.)

63 **Hamiltonian Dynamical Systems: History, Theory, and Applications**
H.S. Dumas, K.R. Meyer, and D.S. Schmidt (eds.)

64 **Systems and Control Theory for Power Systems**
J.H. Chow, P.V. Kokotovic, R.J. Thomas (eds.)

65 **Mathematical Finance**
M.H.A. Davis, D. Duffie, W.H. Fleming, and S.E. Shreve (eds.)

66 **Robust Control Theory** B.A. Francis and P.P. Khargonekar (eds.)

67 **Mathematics in Industrial Problems, Part 7** A. Friedman

68 **Flow Control** M.D. Gunzburger (ed.)

69 **Linear Algebra for Signal Processing**
A. Bojanczyk and G. Cybenko (eds.)
70 **Control and Optimal Design of Distributed Parameter Systems**
J.E. Lagnese, D.L. Russell, and L.W. White (eds.)
71 **Stochastic Networks** F.P. Kelly and R.J. Williams (eds.)
72 **Discrete Probability and Algorithms**
D. Aldous, P. Diaconis, J. Spencer, and J.M. Steele (eds.)
73 **Discrete Event Systems, Manufacturing Systems, and Communication Networks**
P.R. Kumar and P.P. Varaiya (eds.)
74 **Adaptive Control, Filtering, and Signal Processing**
K.J. Åström, G.C. Goodwin, and P.R. Kumar (eds.)
75 **Modeling, Mesh Generation, and Adaptive Numerical Methods for Partial Differential Equations** I. Babuska, J.E. Flaherty, W.D. Henshaw, J.E. Hopcroft, J.E. Oliger, and T. Tezduyar (eds.)
76 **Random Discrete Structures** D. Aldous and R. Pemantle (eds.)
77 **Nonlinear Stochastic PDEs: Hydrodynamic Limit and Burgers' Turbulence** T. Funaki and W.A. Woyczynski (eds.)
78 **Nonsmooth Analysis and Geometric Methods in Deterministic Optimal Control** B.S. Mordukhovich and H.J. Sussmann (eds.)
79 **Environmental Studies: Mathematical, Computational, and Statistical Analysis** M.F. Wheeler (ed.)
80 **Image Models (and their Speech Model Cousins)**
S.E. Levinson and L. Shepp (eds.)
81 **Genetic Mapping and DNA Sequencing**
T. Speed and M.S. Waterman (eds.)
82 **Mathematical Approaches to Biomolecular Structure and Dynamics**
J.P. Mesirov, K. Schulten, and D. Sumners (eds.)
83 **Mathematics in Industrial Problems, Part 8** A. Friedman
84 **Classical and Modern Branching Processes**
K.B. Athreya and P. Jagers (eds.)
85 **Stochastic Models in Geosystems**
S.A. Molchanov and W.A. Woyczynski (eds.)
86 **Computational Wave Propagation**
B. Engquist and G.A. Kriegsmann (eds.)
87 **Progress in Population Genetics and Human Evolution**
P. Donnelly and S. Tavaré (eds.)
88 **Mathematics in Industrial Problems, Part 9** A. Friedman
89 **Multiparticle Quantum Scattering With Applications to Nuclear, Atomic and Molecular Physics** D.G. Truhlar and B. Simon (eds.)
90 **Inverse Problems in Wave Propagation** G. Chavent, G. Papanicolau, P. Sacks, and W.W. Symes (eds.)
91 **Singularities and Oscillations** J. Rauch and M. Taylor (eds.)

92 **Large-Scale Optimization with Applications, Part I: Optimization in Inverse Problems and Design**
L.T. Biegler, T.F. Coleman, A.R. Conn, and F. Santosa (eds.)

93 **Large-Scale Optimization with Applications, Part II: Optimal Design and Control**
L.T. Biegler, T.F. Coleman, A.R. Conn, and F. Santosa (eds.)

94 **Large-Scale Optimization with Applications, Part III: Molecular Structure and Optimization**
L.T. Biegler, T.F. Coleman, A.R. Conn, and F. Santosa (eds.)

95 **Quasiclassical Methods**
J. Rauch and B. Simon (eds.)

96 **Wave Propagation in Complex Media**
G. Papanicolaou (ed.)

97 **Random Sets: Theory and Applications**
J. Goutsias, R.P.S. Mahler, and H.T. Nguyen (eds.)

98 **Particulate Flows: Processing and Rheology**
D.A. Drew, D.D. Joseph, and S.L. Passman (eds.)

99 **Mathematics of Multiscale Materials** K.M. Golden, G.R. Grimmett, R.D. James, G.W. Milton, and P.N. Sen (eds.)

100 **Mathematics in Industrial Problems, Part 10** A. Friedman

101 **Nonlinear Optical Materials** J.V. Moloney (ed.)

102 **Numerical Methods for Polymeric Systems** S.G. Whittington (ed.)

103 **Topology and Geometry in Polymer Science** S.G. Whittington, D. Sumners, and T. Lodge (eds.)

104 **Essays on Mathematical Robotics** J. Baillieul, S.S. Sastry, and H.J. Sussmann (eds.)

105 **Algorithms For Parallel Processing** M.T. Heath, A. Ranade, and R.S. Schreiber (eds.)

106 **Parallel Processing of Discrete Problems** P.M. Pardalos (ed.)

107 **The Mathematics of Information Coding, Extraction, and Distribution** G. Cybenko, D.P. O'Leary, and J. Rissanen (eds.)

108 **Rational Drug Design** D.G. Truhlar, W. Howe, A.J. Hopfinger, J. Blaney, and R.A. Dammkoehler (eds.)

FORTHCOMING VOLUMES

1992–1992: *Control Theory*
Robotics

1996 Summer Program: *Emerging Applications of Number Theory*

1996–1997: *Mathematics in High Performance Computing*
Algorithms for Parallel Processing
Evolutionary Algorithms
The Mathematics of Information Coding, Extraction and Distribution
Structured Adaptive Mesh Refinement Grid Methods
Computational Radiology and Imaging: Therapy and Diagnostics
Mathematical and Computational Issues in Drug Design
Rational Drug Design
Grid Generation and Adaptive Algorithms
Parallel Solution of Partial Differential Equations

1997 Summer Program: *Statistics in the Health Sciences*
Week 1: Genetics
Week 2: Imaging
Week 3: Diagnosis and Prediction
Weeks 4 and 5: Design and Analysis of Clinical Trials
Week 6: Statistics and Epidemiology: Environment and Health

1997–1998: *Emerging Applications for Dynamical Systems*
Numerical Methods for Bifurcation Problems
Multiple-time-scale Dynamical Systems
Dynamics of Algorithms

GPSR Compliance

The European Union's (EU) General Product Safety Regulation (GPSR) is a set of rules that requires consumer products to be safe and our obligations to ensure this.

If you have any concerns about our products, you can contact us on ProductSafety@springernature.com

In case Publisher is established outside the EU, the EU authorized representative is:

Springer Nature Customer Service Center GmbH
Europaplatz 3
69115 Heidelberg, Germany

Batch number: 10704041

Printed by Printforce, the Netherlands